FROM PANIC TO POTENTIAL

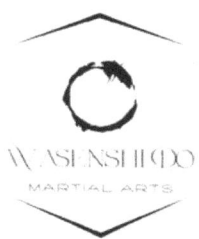

By Farren Segura Tayler

Copyright © 2025 Farren Segura Tayler

All rights reserved. No part of this publication may be reproduced, distributed, or transmitted in any form or by any means, including photocopying, recording, or other electronic or mechanical methods, without the prior written permission of the publisher, except in the case of brief quotations embodied in critical reviews and certain other noncommercial uses permitted by copyright law. For permission requests, write to the publisher, addressed "Attention: Permissions Coordinator." at the address below.

JSBN: 9798218788933 (Paperback)
ISBN- 9798218788926 (eBook)

Any references to historical events, real people, or real places are used fictitiously. Names, characters, and places are products of the author's imagination.

Book design by Farren Segura Tayler

Printed by IngramSpark - in the United States of America.

First printing edition 2025.

Wasenshido Ryu LLC
Connecticut 06035

www.Wasenshido.com
www.FromPanicToPotential.com
www.YogiWarriors.org

"This book is sincerely dedicated to my perfect, beautiful, loving, funny, wholesome, honest, intelligent, sweet, caring wife, without whom this book would not have been possible."

Presented by Farren Segura Tayler and Wasenshi Do Ryu Martial Arts

Farren is not just a world traveler. He's a seeker, health coach, martial arts coach, functional nutrition and wellness enthusiast, Qigong practitioner and certified Yoga instructor. Farren has a deep passion for coaching people in their transformation. For the past 25 years, Farren has journeyed across continents, tirelessly dedicating himself to his personal healing odyssey. Through over two decades of self-study in functional and integrative approaches to health, I've applied these principles in my own life and shared them with clients."

He's explored the depths of both alternative medicine, nutrition science, modern western psychology, such as Cognitive Behavioral Therapy, and delved into ancient practices and modern therapies in search of true wellness and longevity. It's been his insatiable quest, and now he wants to share what he's learned with you.

What you hold in your hands is more than just a book—it's a guide crafted from decades of experience, hard–earned wisdom, and a relentless pursuit of inner peace and fulfillment. In these pages, Farren shares the secrets he's uncovered on his path, which has led him to a healthier and more peaceful way of living. This is a path that you too can follow.

This book is an invitation to embark on your own journey towards a life of balance, purpose, and profound fulfillment. Whether you're seeking physical well–being, mental clarity, or spiritual awakening, this book offers a roadmap to help get you there.

Farren's story is proof that transformation is possible and that healing is within reach. A life of peace and purpose is not just a dream, but a reality waiting for you to claim. *"From Panic to Potential"* is your guide to live a life without chronic pain, panic and excessive anxiety.

Welcome to your new beginning.

"Everyone has the potential to be better than they were yesterday."

It's a really good quality, to be able to find the treasure within the suffering, but it doesn't mean the treasure is the destination."
— Farren Segura Tayler

Waiver and Release

The information provided in *"From Panic to Potential"* by Farren Segura Tayler (the "Author") is for general informational and educational purposes only.

While the content in this book is provided in good faith, it does not constitute professional medical advice, diagnosis, or treatment. Always seek the advice of a qualified healthcare provider with any questions you may have regarding any medical condition or mental health concern.

The Author does not guarantee the accuracy, relevance, timeliness, or completeness of any information on these topics. The information presented in this book is not intended to replace or countermand medical or psychological advice offered by physicians, therapists, or other licensed healthcare providers.

The Author shall not be liable for any direct, indirect, consequential, special, exemplary, or any other damages of any kind arising from the use of this book, including, but not limited to, economic loss, injury, illness, or death. You, the Reader, are reading and using this information at your own risk.

The use of information from *"From Panic to Potential"* is strictly voluntary and at the Reader's sole risk. The Author does not recommend or endorse any specific tests, physicians, practitioners, teachers, products, procedures, opinions, or other information that may be mentioned in the book. Reliance on any information provided by this book is solely at your own risk.

IMPORTANT NOTE:
Please be aware that working through the material in this book may bring up feelings of anxiety, unresolved trauma, or healing symptoms, including paradoxical reactions where things may feel more intense before they get better. This is a normal part of deep healing work. Take it slow, honor your own pace, and seek professional support if needed. This guide is based on my own lived experience, as well as the insights of many doctors and experts—some of whom have worked with hundreds or even thousands of clients in this field. Use this material as a supportive companion, not as a replacement for professional care.

This program/book/course includes discussions of trauma, post-traumatic stress disorder ("PTSD"), panic, anxiety, and emotional dysregulation. Some content may bring up distressing memories or emotions. Please proceed with care and prioritize your well-being.

If you experience overwhelming emotions, panic, shortness of breath, wheezing, chest tightness, or a sense of constricted airways, stop immediately and seek medical attention. These may be signs of a serious medical issue. Call 911 or go to the nearest emergency room or urgent care center.

This material is intended for educational and informational purposes only. It is not a substitute for medical, psychological, or emergency care. Always consult with a licensed healthcare professional before starting or modifying any wellness program.

By reading this book, you hereby release and discharge the Author from any and all liability and/or responsibility for any and all legal, health, financial, emotional, mental, and/or other personal or non-personal matters.

TABLE OF CONTENTS

Preface 2
Introduction 4
Acknowledgment and Compassion 10
Knowledge and Awareness: 22
To Know and Understand 22
Nutrition and Supplementation: 62
Doctor, Doctor Give Me the News 116
Signs, Symptoms and Sensations of Panic and Anxiety 132
The Breath 166
Cognitive Behavior Therapy 180
Yoga – Rise Up and Out of Your Shell 230
QiGong – Embodiment and Feeling Safe 258
Nature, Exercise and Martial Arts 286
The Story of Your Life 306
Suggested Experts & Resources 346

Preface

I feel like a walking miracle—not because of a sudden miraculous cure, but because of the extraordinary blessings and unwavering support I've received over the years. My journey from the depths of despair, chronic PTSD, daily panic 'attacks,' to the heights of personal achievement has been marked by incredible highs and devastating lows. There were moments when I was on the brink of losing everything, from periods of homelessness to isolation and loneliness, when it felt like there was no one to turn to for support.

In the following pages, I share the story of my transformation. From where I started to where I am now, my journey is a testament to resilience and the power of hope. My hope is that my story will inspire you to find your own strength, no matter the challenges you face.

The world can be an incredible playground of unimaginable success and happiness. But it can also be a tough, stressful place to navigate. From global pandemics and political turmoil to the pressures of social media, job insecurity, and personal relationships, the sources of stress and anxiety seem endless. Yet, even in the midst of all this, there is hope, and there is a way forward. Some sources of stress are glaring and unavoidable, while others hum quietly in the background, subtly but steadily chipping away at our peace of mind. But all of them can be debilitating, leaving us feeling overwhelmed and lost.

It doesn't have to be this way. Let's embark on a journey together to shed the burdens we carry and discover a path to peace and resilience. Together, we can create a brighter future where we support and uplift each other and transform our struggles into stepping stones toward a better life.

My goal is to help you live in a body that feels safe, and to reclaim a sense of security and well-being that may have been lost along the way. This book is designed to teach your brain, mind and body that trauma no longer needs to define you and that healing is possible, within reach, accessible and livable. I have an insatiable drive and thirst for growth and transformation. In my pursuit of ultimate health and longevity, as it's been my scholarly obsession, I hope that this book helps you truly in any way.

This book has been more than seven years in the making. I truly believe it's something special, and I'm proud, not just of the final result, but of the entire process, those who helped in the creation, and what it took to complete it.

So, take this journey for a healthier, happier life, and step into a future where you feel empowered, resilient, and truly alive.

Introduction

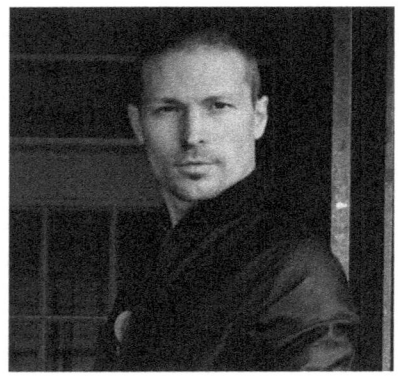

I'm Farren, and I'm truly honored to be here with you. Before we dive into this journey together, I want to share a bit of my story with you because I believe that my experiences can be a guiding force for you, especially if you're living with post–traumatic stress disorder ("PTSD") chronic illness, panic, pain, anxiety, depression or any other host of disabilities or issues.

From a very young age, I faced the challenges of panic and anxiety. By the time I was just 8 years old, these struggles became a constant part of my life. For over 30 years, I endured relentless panic attacks. Until my mid–30s, these attacks were a shadow that followed me everywhere. I never took anything to help during these events. When I was young, my main stress response was to *freeze*. Freeze is one of the three stress responses, the other two being *fight or flight*. Most people have one main response, but I would also have *flight or flee*. This built the base for the psychological trauma that would plague me for the next few decades.

I also experienced an intense, debilitating chronic illness, panic and anxiety, and physical pain throughout my body, which began when I was around seven or eight years old and persisted for almost three decades. I found myself living in my car for weeks on end, feeling isolated and alone, contributing to my depression and anxiety.

Eventually, I reached a point in life where anger, exhaustion, and depression took hold of me. I felt lethargic, apathetic, and numb. I was overwhelmed by sadness, helplessness, hopelessness, and fear. Every corner I turned seemed to be filled with new fears. Yes, there were good times, moments of joy and high spirits, but they were always overshadowed by a storm that was always on the horizon and close by.

I often found myself spiraling downward, struggling just to keep my head above water. I was trapped in a cycle of negative patterns that I couldn't seem to escape. The pain even became so intense that there were times I could barely walk. I couldn't hold down a job because of the constant physical and emotional turmoil. It was a dark time to say the least.

But here's the truth: I've been where you are, and I've come through to the other side. Today, I no longer experience chronic physical pain. I no longer live in the grip of chronic anxiety. I no longer suffer from panic attacks. There is hope, and there is a way out. If I can find peace and healing, so can you. Because in spite of these challenges, I accomplished some incredible things in life. I've walked the path of struggle and hardship, and I've come out on the other side stronger and more resilient. My hope is that by sharing my journey, I can help you navigate your own challenges to find the peace and strength you deserve.

My journey really started when I left my small town in Wisconsin when I was 22 years old with a dream of becoming a martial artist on the big screen, pursuing a full-time career in martial arts. I did end up on the big screen for three hundred million people in China to see. Filming a little show called "KungFu Star – Global Competition." Little did I know that this journey would become the beginning of my healing journey, the path that would transform my life in ways I never imagined. I know that might sound a little cheesy or cliché but, it's true. From that moment on, I dedicated myself to growth, self–discovery, self–mastery and healing. I was thirsty for it, a relentless seeker who couldn't get enough.

Along my path, I was blessed to learn from an incredible array of teachers and healers. I met shamans, yogis, healers, medicine people, mountain people, chiropractors, western doctors, mediums, clairvoyants, psychologists, Master martial artist and more. I began experimenting with natural medicines, trying anything that could offer relief and healing. I was desperate but determined. Each lesson, each experience, helped me move forward, leveling up in my understanding and my healing.

I began to build a toolbox of powerful techniques and wisdom—tools that have guided me on my journey and continue to do so. Now I feel a deep passion for helping, guiding, and coaching others on their own paths. There's nothing more fulfilling than helping someone improve their life, no matter how big or small the change is. It's the greatest feeling in the world, and it's why I'm here. I want to share what I've learned and to be a guiding light for others on their own path to healing and growth.

In this book, you will embark on a transformative journey of understanding, growth, and healing. Each chapter is designed to guide you deeper into your own self–discovery, and to help you unlock the strength, resilience, and peace that lies within you. You'll learn to navigate the complexities of your mind and body and emerge with a renewed sense of purpose and clarity. This journey isn't just about gaining knowledge; it's about experiencing real, tangible change in your life. It's about shedding old patterns that no longer serve you and stepping into a life that feels authentic, empowered, and fulfilling.

Before we dive any deeper, I want to make something clear: I'm not claiming to be an expert in every subject covered in this book. I'm not a doctor, therapist, or licensed professional, at least not in the conventional sense. What I *am* is someone who's lived this. These pages reflect my story, my healing journey, and the countless hours I've spent studying, researching, and testing various tools, techniques, and methods, many of which have truly changed my life. I've taken what's worked for me and started sharing it with close friends and family, helping them through their own struggles. And now, as I begin to work with private clients, I've seen how powerful these approaches can be when tailored to real people dealing with real challenges.

This book isn't a collection of textbook definitions or theory. It's a practical, lived experience woven together with research, curiosity, and a deep desire to heal—not just myself, but to help others find their own way out of pain, confusion, anxiety, and chronic illness. I invite you to read it with an open mind and an open heart. Take what resonates, leave what doesn't, and use this as a guide—not a prescription—for your own adventure of Life.

This book is designed for those who are ready to go beyond conventional treatment alone and are committed to addressing what I believe are the root causes of panic, anxiety, and chronic disorders. Whether you're currently on medication, considering it, or pursuing other forms of care, everything in this book is intended to support and complement your healing journey, not compete with it. This approach is especially crafted for individuals who are introspective, motivated to deepen their self-awareness, and ready to break free from the cycles of panic and chronic pain.

This is my mission: to share the wisdom I've gathered and, through this book and the other ways I support others, help you become the best version of yourself. Together, we'll uncover the tools you need to heal, grow, and thrive.

The following is a list of many of the things that I've studied and implemented and that benefited myself and what I use to help others:

- Martial Arts
- Nutrition, wellness, biohacking and lifestyle changes
- Yoga (I have my 200 RYT from HIBS Yoga)
- Various styles of pranayama (breathwork)
- Qigong – medical qigong
- Chinese medicine – meridian therapy
- Knowledge and wisdom from acupuncture
- Vitamin and mineral supplementation

- Various forms of energetic healing
- Vagus nerve therapy
- Thai massage - Tuina – Somatic techniques
- Neuro Linguistic Programming (language and sensory technique that helps change thoughts and behavior)
- Coffee enema therapy
- Fasting – liver cleansing
- Physical therapy/ mobility – exercise
- Emotion code
- Cognitive Behavior Therapy ("CBT") – Western psychology
- Emotional Freedom Technique ("EFT")
- GAPS – Gut and Psychological/Physiological symptoms Diet
- Ketogenic diet with intermittent fasting
- Carnivore diet
- Nature bathing and Grounding
- Meditation
- Wisdom of the 5 elements – earth – air – water – fire – ethereal
- Ancient wisdom and knowledge

Who is this book for?
- Anyone and Everyone!
- If you want to learn more about yourself and have more self–awareness
- You've experienced a panic attack.
- You've experienced anxiety—mild or intense.
- You live with chronic pain or persistent physical symptoms.
- You feel stuck or stagnant, no matter what you try.
- Fear or constant worry is your baseline.
- Depression weighs on your heart and mind.
- You've felt helpless, hopeless, or unsure of how to move forward.
- You battle self–sabotage or patterns that hold you back.
- You feel exhausted, drained, or chronically fatigued.
- You generally feel unwell in life and need support

If even one of these resonates with you, this book can serve as a guide to help you navigate your way toward healing, strength, and clarity.

What you'll need to begin:
- Just show up as you are.
- Try to have an open mind, willing to explore new ideas and practices.
- *Optional:* A notebook and pen to capture insights or patterns.
- *Optional:* A journal to track your progress. Personally, I like to use a digital journal with titles like *"From Panic to Potential"* or something empowering and personal like *"No longer will I live like this."*

Chapter 1
Acknowledgment and Compassion

"Healing doesn't mean the damage never existed. It means the damage no longer controls our lives."
— Akshay Dubey

One of the most powerful things someone ever told me was, "it's okay to feel this way." In that moment, I didn't feel particularly okay. But this acknowledgment and willingness to see me as I was, meant everything.

I want you to know that experiencing anxiety or panic is not a sign of weakness, but a testament to your strength. Going through anxiety and panic shows your capacity to feel deeply and carry those emotions, even when they seem overwhelming. Vulnerability is not a weakness.

I like to think of it this way: you might be someone who feels things strongly, deeply, and empathetically. That's a gift. For me, being a "feeling" person means I experience and feel emotions more intensely and deeply than most. Sometimes a beautiful piece of music can send chills through my body, filling me with joy. Other times, I might be overcome with emotions like sadness, guilt, or despair, with tears streaming down my face. But whether the emotions are positive or challenging, they remind me that I'm alive, deeply connected to the world around me, and that is something powerful.

Life can also feel like a relentless cycle of ups and downs, a pattern that often accompanies anxiety and depression. There are moments when I find myself trapped in a state of worry and fear, diving too deeply into those thoughts. This usually leads to a downward spiral. The reason I bring these ideas to light is to raise awareness. When it comes to panic and anxiety, or a panic situation, those of us who feel deeply and are sensitive to emotions like fear, worry, and angst, are more easily triggered into anxious states. This also usually means, people with a past of trauma.

The first step is simply recognizing this pattern. Awareness is key. We'll explore this more deeply in the CBT chapter, but for now, I want to ask you: are you someone who feels deeply and empathetically toward others and the world around you?

Now, one of the most comforting things anyone ever told me was, "You're not alone in this." At first, I had a strange thought: how selfish am I to think I'm the only one going through this? The truth is, many people in today's world are dealing with the same struggles, each in their own unique way. Statistics show that millions of people experience panic situations. So, take a deep breath and remind yourself: you're not alone in this. Others are going through this too, and there is support.

You are not weak. Sometimes being overwhelmed is a sign of just how strong you are to have taken on so much in life. But even the strongest need to take a step back, breathe, and seek support. You are resilient, and you are not alone.

I used to think there was something "wrong" with me. But let me tell you, that's absolutely not true—not for me back then, and not for you now. The belief that "I'm not good enough" or "there's something wrong with me" is one of the most common and crippling limiting beliefs that many of us carry. But these are just lies we tell ourselves that become the chain that holds us back from living fully and freely. Try not to compare yourself to others. Some people are made different, not better. Others may be able to handle certain circumstances better than you can and that's ok. You are not meant to be everything to everyone and be everything to the world and do everything all the time and be perfect and so on and so forth. This can cause a lot of stress and after a long time, PTSD. You have certain skills and talents that are different than others. This can be a factor in the way we live our lives and create unnecessary stress.

I know what it's like to feel stuck and to feel like everything you do is shrouded in fear. Even the simplest tasks, like driving across town on the highway, felt terrifying to me. I'd stick to the side roads just to feel safe. I was even scared to leave town, go for a hike, or be in social gatherings. I was even scared to get the help I desperately needed because I feared having another panic situation. I felt like I was constantly balancing on a double-edged sword. But guess what? There is a way out, my friend.

For most of my life, I've had this strange but powerful image in my mind. I saw myself as a person trapped in a deep cave, chained to the floor, but with a light shining down on me from above. I felt stuck, unable to reach that light. But the truth is that the light was and is within my reach. And it is in your reach too. What I have to share with you in this book can help you break those chains and step into the light of your own life.

Throughout these pages, I'll explain certain concepts many times over because I want you to truly grasp and fully understand what's happening in your mind and body. Together, we'll unravel the mysteries of anxiety, fear, and limiting beliefs. Together, we'll find the way out.

Despite how far we've come, there remains this common misconception that dealing with PTSD, trauma, anxiety, and similar challenges is a sign of weakness. I want to take a moment to break down this stigma. Imagine a soldier returning from war with PTSD. This soldier is someone who was resilient, fit, strong, and disciplined. Are they now weak because they've experienced horrific trauma? Absolutely not. It's not about being strong or weak; it's about how trauma is processed in the brain, mind and body and how we work through it.

This concept is crucial to understand, and as you read through these pages, you'll see why. We'll dive into the reasons why trauma affects people differently and what can be done about it. Two people might go through the same traumatic experience. Yet one might seem to move on without issue, while the other develops PTSD. What's the difference? The answer isn't simple, but one likely reason is that the person with PTSD may have unresolved childhood trauma or a brain that processes stimuli in a way that makes them more vulnerable to the effects of trauma. This combination can create a perfect storm, leading to PTSD. Another difference may be that one soldier returning home may have more support in family, friends and sense of purpose while another soldier might come home to nothing, a spouse that left them, etc. Which one do you think might develop PTSD more so than the other? The one with less support of course. This doesn't mean everyone in the same situation as the less supported soldier is more likely to develop PTSD, but studies have shown that a support system can reduce the likelihood of developing PTSD.

> **IMPORTANT NOTE:**
> Nutritional deficiencies and "Gut Dysbiosis" play an important role in a dysregulated nervous system, causing hormonal and chemical imbalances in the body, brain, and nervous system. This can make it harder for you to manage your symptoms. *See* Chapter 3 for more information.

This book is here to help you understand these complexities and guide you toward healing. Keep reading to learn more about how trauma works and, more importantly, how you can work through it. The journey to understanding and healing is within reach, and we'll navigate it together.

We must take responsibility for our own well–being. This might sound like a daunting task, especially when life throws challenges our way. The weight of our work, relationships, health, and personal growth can sometimes feel overwhelming. However, taking responsibility for our well–being isn't about carrying the weight of the world on our shoulders alone. In fact, it's quite the opposite.

Taking responsibility means recognizing that we have the power to shape our lives, and with that power comes the ability to seek out and accept help. The beautiful truth is that we are never truly alone on this journey. There is an abundance of support available to us and embracing that support is a crucial part of taking responsibility for our well-being. If accepting help is a triggering area for you, this is something to think about when you get to Chapter 7 on Cognitive Behavior.

Imagine your life as a journey and on this journey, you're carrying a backpack filled with your experiences, emotions, and challenges. Sometimes that backpack feels too heavy to bear. But what if I told you that along the path, there are countless people who are willing to help lighten your load? All you need to do is reach out, ask for help, and allow them to support you.

THERE IS NO SHAME IN SEEKING SUPPORT. It's a sign of strength and self–awareness. We are not meant to do everything ALL alone ALL the time. Whether it's talking to a trusted friend, working with a therapist, or engaging in self–care practices like meditation, exercise, or journaling, these are all ways of taking responsibility for your well–being. You are acknowledging that while you are in charge of your life, you don't have to do it all alone.

The resources available today are vast and varied. Help is everywhere from online communities that provide connection and understanding, to books and courses that offer guidance and knowledge. There are also professionals like therapists, coaches, and doctors who are dedicated to helping you navigate your challenges. Help is even in the words of a supportive friend, on the advice of a wise mentor, and in the tools and techniques shared in this book.

Taking responsibility for your well–being also means setting boundaries, knowing your limits, and giving yourself permission to rest when you need it. It's about understanding that you are worthy of care, both from yourself and from others. Sometimes, taking responsibility means saying "no" to the things that drain you and "yes" to the things that nourish your mind, body and soul.

It's important to remember that this responsibility is not about perfection. It's about progress. It's about making small, intentional choices each day that move you closer to the life you want to live. It's about being kind to yourself when you stumble, and knowing that every step forward, no matter how small, is a victory.

So, as you continue on your journey, remember that taking responsibility for your well-being is not a solitary endeavor. It's about embracing the support around you, recognizing your own worth, and making choices that honor your health, happiness, and growth. The road ahead may have its challenges, but with the help available to you, it's a road you don't have to walk alone. You have the power to shape your life, and there are countless hands ready to help guide you along the way.

IMPORTANT NOTE:
One of the techniques that has helped provide me with immediate relief is EFT (Emotional Freedom Technique). The EFT technique I use is the one taught and demonstrated by Brad Yates. He teaches EFT free on his YouTube channel. I recommend searching "EFT for panic with Brad Yates" on YouTube and use it anytime you feel a panic situation coming up. When I felt a panic attack coming on, I would immediately go to one of his videos and I would feel a huge relief sometimes even within 1 minute! I wanted to share this as one of the first things in the book as it was so immediately helpful and supportive for me and so many others.

EFT – What is it Exactly?

EFT is a powerful, holistic technique designed to help you overcome trauma, PTSD, fears, and various mental and physical challenges. This technique uniquely combines the ancient wisdom of Chinese medicine with modern therapeutic practices by using your fingertips to tap on specific acupressure points on your body.

EFT is a transformative practice that empowers you to manage and control your emotions, thoughts, and feelings. The fundamental principle behind EFT is that negative, traumatic, or intrusive thoughts disrupt the delicate balance of your nervous system. By tapping on key areas of your body while consciously reframing these thoughts, you can restore equilibrium, bringing both your mind and body back into harmony.

While I won't be teaching the EFT technique in detail within this book, you'll find that following along with video demonstrations is more than sufficient to learn and apply EFT effectively. These videos will guide you step–by–step to make it easy to incorporate EFT into your daily routine and experience its profound benefits. Through this simple yet powerful technique, you'll have the ability to release the emotional burdens that have been holding you back and step into a life of greater peace, freedom, and emotional well–being.

Living with PTSD and chronic illness doesn't just impact the individual—its effects ripple outward, touching loved ones, friends, and even colleagues. In my own experience, my struggles with trauma and health challenges created significant stress and confusion for those around me. Loved ones often carry a heavy emotional load, worrying about your well–being, feeling helpless, and sometimes experiencing frustration when they're unsure how to support you. Friends might become distant or cautious, unsure how to interact or fearful of causing further distress. At work, colleagues may misinterpret fatigue or emotional reactivity, leading to misunderstandings or strained relationships. I've observed similar patterns in others close to me who deal with chronic conditions or trauma; relationships can feel strained, and communication can become challenging. Recognizing this ripple effect is crucial—not only for your healing journey but for fostering empathy and openness, helping those around you understand and support your path toward recovery.

Improving these situations begins with clear, open, and honest communication. It's essential to educate those around you about your experience and limitations, helping them understand that your behaviors or reactions are symptoms, not personal choices. Setting healthy boundaries, expressing gratitude, and clearly sharing what support looks like for you can significantly ease tension. Encouraging loved ones to learn about your condition, perhaps through books, articles, or support groups, can also foster empathy and deepen connection. Remember, nurturing these relationships through patience, compassion, and communication creates a foundation of mutual understanding and resilience.

I want to take a moment here to talk to any and all veterans reading my book:

Thank you for your service and thank you for taking the time to read this. I was never a veteran. I don't know what it feels like to go into the military, serving your country, coming home, or back to society with some or any form of trauma. Not to mention any injuries sustained and other emotional troubles. I will say PTSD and C-PTSD are all intertwined and connected. You are NOT weak or frail or a victim to these symptoms you're feeling. PERIOD. Yes, they are part of your life, yes, you feel them, and yes, they suck; I'll give you that. It's a horrible feeling, and it can be incapacitating. This is where we have to be courageous and stronger than those symptoms. Getting help doesn't mean that you've succumbed to this terrible feeling or feelings. It doesn't mean you are any less of a man, or woman or person. If you're a man reading this, to me it's the most powerful masculine action to stand the hell up and say, screw this, I'm going to take action, make it a mission to fix this! Make it a mission, if you choose to accept it, soldier. Sounds a little cheesy, but I'm very serious. This is your life here, your family, your career, your livelihood.

I will say you do need some help if you live with C-PTSD or other challenges like depression or other disorders. I had a lot of help, no one does anything by themselves. The most badass Special Forces teams rely on each other to complete missions. Arnold Schwarzenegger, one of the most badass men ever, says he himself had a lot of help and was absolutely not a self-made man. The list goes on with very successful women and men that needed help and support to overcome adversity and be who they are. We all do. In the next few chapters well go into more about symptoms and what your body may be telling you.

The knowledge, exercises and techniques in this book will fully apply to you and anyone with these symptoms. I did join a martial arts boot camp scenario where I moved and lived in the camp while training and studying for many years. My teacher at the time previously trained Special Forces teams so we got a little of that training as well. I felt part of something bigger than me and larger than life. After years of that, I struggled to transition back into society, which came with depression, anxiety and recurrence of C-PTSD (complex) symptoms.

A lot of these techniques in this book have been used to help veterans with PTSD and other emotional trauma, including depression. Emotional Freedom Technique (EFT) and Cognitive Behavior Therapy (CBT) are two in particular. I do mention EFT and point you to an expert that I used and has helped me greatly. We go into more detail about CBT in Chapter 7. Your nervous system is dis-regulated. Let's get that back in complete working order so you can move forward with your life. You're now debriefed and ready to take the next necessary steps.

IMPORTANT NOTE:
IF YOU HAVE SUICIDAL OR OTHER HARMFUL THOUGHTS – NEVER FORGET THAT YOU'RE WORTH IT, YOU CAN LIVE A HAPPY HEALTHY LIFE, IT JUST MAY TAKE TIME AND SOME HARD WORK.

IF YOU OR SOMEONE YOU KNOW HAS SUICIDAL THOUGHTS, GET HELP RIGHT AWAY.

Ways to help or get help:
- Call 911 for a wellness check
- Reach out to a close friend or loved one.
- Contact a minister, spiritual leader, or someone in your faith community.
- Contact a suicide hotline.
    - In the U.S., call or text 988 to reach the 988 Suicide & Crisis Lifeline, available 24 hours a day, seven days a week. Or use the Lifeline Chat. Services are free and confidential.
    - U.S. veterans or service members who are in crisis can call 988 and then press "1" for the Veterans Crisis Line. Or text 838255. Or chat online.
    - The Suicide & Crisis Lifeline in the U.S. has a Spanish language phone line at 1–888–628–9454 (toll–free).
- Make an appointment with your healthcare professional or mental health professional.

When to get emergency help:

IF YOU THINK YOU MAY HURT YOURSELF OR ATTEMPT SUICIDE, CALL 911 OR YOUR LOCAL EMERGENCY NUMBER RIGHT AWAY.

If you know someone who's in danger of attempting suicide or has made a suicide attempt, make sure someone stays with that person for safety. Call 911 or your local emergency number right away. Or, if you can do so safely, take the person to the nearest hospital emergency department.

When to see a doctor:

Chapter 4 is where I go into detail on this. Talk to your healthcare professional or a mental health professional if you have disturbing thoughts and feelings about a traumatic event for more than a month, especially if they're severe. Also, see a health professional if you're having trouble getting your life back under control. Getting treatment as soon as possible can help prevent PTSD symptoms from getting worse.

Takeaways from Chapter 1

- It's okay to feel this way right now. Seriously—it is. You may wish you felt different, and that's exactly why you're here: because you're ready for change. That alone says a lot about your strength.
- If you're experiencing anxiety, panic, or emotional overwhelm, you may be dealing with a dysregulated nervous system. This book will walk you through exactly what that means and offer tools to help bring your system back into balance.
- Let's get something straight: anxiety or panic is *not* a sign of weakness. Period.
- Some people feel the world more deeply—it's just how certain brains are wired. If that sounds like you, welcome to the club. It's not a flaw; it's part of your design.
- Spoiler alert: you're not alone.
- You're not broken. Your nervous system and body might just be a bit dysregulated, but that's why you're here.
- And there *is* a way out of this.
- You're not wrong, bad, or backwards, so let's put that false story to rest.
- Yes, it's up to us to take responsibility for our own well–being—but the good news? You don't have to do it alone. There is so much support, information, and healing available once you know where to look.
- Lastly, remember this: PTSD and chronic illness can deeply impact those around you, too. Friends, partners, family, and coworkers might not fully understand what it feels like to live in your world. That's okay. Just stay open, educate when you can, and be gentle with both yourself and others along the way.
- I hope you'll stick with me through to the very last chapter where I bring everything we've covered together into clear, easy-to-digest steps designed to inspire real, lasting change.

Chapter 2
Knowledge and Awareness:
To Know and Understand

"The body keeps the score. If the mind won't let it speak, the body will."
— Bessel van der Kolk

What IS panic? What IS anxiety? What IS stress? Each of these can mean different things for different people. But let's get straight into how I've come to learn what these terms mean. In this second chapter, I want to be clear that my goal is to keep things simple—just a bird's-eye view to help you ease in. We'll go deeper into the details as the book unfolds.

Breaking Down and Defining "Panic"

In its simplest terms, panic is your body "over responding" to something that it thinks is dangerous, throwing you into a fight or flight response. I want you to keep in mind that there is a difference between a real threat and a perceived threat. This is common sense to our conscious minds, but sometimes our subconscious or the unconscious part of us doesn't realize the difference, and we have to remind ourselves that there is a difference.

A real threat is a tiger chasing you, getting attacked in an alleyway, or someone breaking into your house. In these scenarios, people will most likely have a fight or flight response where adrenaline will kick in and flow into your blood. Blood will then flow more into the muscles for running or fighting, and non–survival systems shut down, such as the immune and digestive systems. This is also called hypervigilance. This is when someone is extremely alert and constantly looking for potential threats or dangers, even when there's no immediate reason to be afraid.

It's like being in a state of heightened awareness all the time, where your senses are always "on edge," making you overly cautious or anxious, even in safe situations. It's often linked to stress, trauma, or anxiety, and it can be mentally exhausting because you're always on the lookout for something bad to happen. These are great lifesaving responses that we all have, and they are normal responses for us. But it's when our bodies and minds perceive danger that isn't really there that issues start to arise.

I'm going to share with you an analogy about how I best understand panic, which has helped me greatly in my life. Think of the toaster in your kitchen. Let's say you're using this toaster and it's working properly. The toast pops up just like you want it to, because you set it to pop up with the perfect brown crisp you like. Everything is in working order. What if this toaster for "some reason" happens to NOT pop up when it's supposed to and it starts to burn your toast? Smoke comes out of the top and sets off the fire alarm. This setting of the fire alarm is analogous to a "panic attack." Michael from *PanicFree TV*, called this the panic "false alarm." This was HUGE for me in my understanding and my overcoming panic.

I thought to myself, "so this panic is what happens when my body over responds or overreacts to something??" This then ties into PTSD because every time the "false alarm" goes off, my body would go into panic mode, even when there wasn't anything really happening. In other words, for an irrational reason. From there, I was able to start using the tools I had, to start digging for clues as to why this reaction was happening. Just knowing and understanding this can be a huge help and create more calm. It definitely was for me! Another way to look at this is that after years of feeling irrational danger, your body and mind become hyper focused and used to the feeling. You start to have a short fuse to anything resembling danger and to any triggers you may have.

I went through the mindset at one point and thought, "isn't my body intelligent enough to know the difference and this is all just happening for some deeper reason?" The short answer is no. The body is an amazing, advanced machine. It's mechanical in a sense and it has an intelligence that it knows what to do to keep us as balanced, healthy as possible and in homeostasis. This is coming from someone that has always and will always be in the search for the core deeper meaning, root causes of things as much as I can. I needed to bring that into balance, swing the lever the other direction a little to find balance. Western psychology is what really brought me more into balance in my life.

Another point I want to share is that in this new era we live in, starting with social media and the internet and technology boom, there is this whole world that is new to us. So much subconscious baggage can be created from diving into things like social media that can create angst and depression. It can ALSO create amazing opportunities and can change your life for the better! Technology and social media are amazing tools and creative outlets when used in a positive way.

But when we are surrounded by so many electronics and stimuli from TV, phones, social media, computers, and advertisements, all of that can overwhelm us. If we're not solid and comfortable within ourselves, we can get caught up in the world of emotions. We look at Facebook or Instagram and we judge ourselves, create jealousy, get angry at each other, and see too many depressing things etc. Too many impressions can overwhelm us, cause us to spiral emotionally, create stress. List goes on.

Sometimes there are those that if they don't go back out to nature and connect, go on a hike, go into the woods to reconnect, or ground and balance out because they are so caught up in the online world. We can then feel out of whack or discombobulated if you will. When you feel stressed out, you need to find relaxation and peace.

Let's recap

As I told you in Chapter 1, you are not wrong, bad, weak, backwards, or anything like that. So many people across the globe are affected by panic, anxiety, and stress every day. AND there can be good reasons for this. BUT don't get this mixed up with the idea that people with PTSD and panic disorder don't have their own good reasons. It's just that their nervous systems have become dysregulated, meaning it's not functioning naturally anymore, so panic and anxiety become the default hypervigilant state. This is when you need to learn how to bring the body back to homeostasis, back to BALANCE. That's what this book is for!

Let's look at some of the reasons someone may experience anxiety, stress or panic symptoms:
- SOCIAL MEDIA
- Triggered responses from past trauma (PTSD)
- Being overwhelmed – burned out
- Being overworked
- Feeling scattered in too many directions
- Stress
- Survival needs are not being met
- Loss of a job
- Lack of financial security
- Health problems
- Aging
- Relationship challenges
- Depression
- Limiting beliefs and limited belief systems
- Unreasonable expectations
- Stuck emotions in the body
- Food allergies
- Grief, fear, anxiety and other dysregulated emotions, worsening your symptoms
- The future of society or humanity
- Feelings of regret or other things from the past

All these things, these natural stressors, are all part of normal existence. But some people experience these things more than others and some of these things are worse in certain areas.

Throughout this book, we will investigate how to deal with these situations, and not just to learn how to cope with them, but to learn real healing and empowering ways for you to live a happier, healthier, and more abundant life. This is a right we are all entitled to.

I want to now address an important emotion: anger. You might already be dealing with anger, or you may have shoved it under the rug so to speak. Anger is an emotion that often doesn't get enough attention when we talk about anxiety and depression, yet it's deeply connected to both. Anger is like a hidden storm within us, building up over time and, if left unaddressed, it contributes to the very anxiety we're trying to manage.

When anger and frustration are bottled up, they create an imbalance within us, disrupting the flow of energy through our bodies. This disruption affects our meridians (channels of how our energy flows), organs, joints, and more. Stagnant energy can lead to stagnant blood flow, which, in turn, can "suffocate" our organs and slow down our metabolism. When our metabolism suffers, so do our mitochondria—the powerhouses of our cells. Mitochondrial dysfunction is linked to nearly every disease and disorder in the body, including mental health challenges. The connection is clear: our emotions, particularly unresolved anger and others, have a direct impact on our physical health.

It's important to understand that feeling anger and frustration is completely normal. What matters is how we choose to express these emotions. Finding healthy outlets is key—exercise, yoga, or having an honest conversation with the person who contributed to those feelings can all be powerful ways to release anger. Even talking to someone you trust or seeking support from a therapist can make a world of difference.

As we explore this theme further, let's not forget the importance of compassion and understanding, especially towards ourselves. Much of this work is about healing our inner child, the parts of us that still carry wounds from childhood and adolescence. But it's also about recognizing that we have to become fully responsible for our own wellbeing. We must become our own parent, set healthy boundaries and practice self–discipline.

Again, there is so much support available—like this book and countless other resources and professionals. Give yourself permission to take in this new knowledge and information but also be ready to push yourself forward. Start your healing journey today, and watch your life transform before your eyes. The power to change is within you, and it starts with acknowledging and honoring your emotions, including anger, as part of your path to wholeness.

PANIC TO POTENTIAL QUESTION:
Why did I feel fine when I was younger, but now that I'm older those old wounds keep resurfacing and triggering so much stress?

The answer to this lies in how our bodies and minds manage stress and trauma over time. When we're younger, we tend to be more resilient. Our bodies and minds have a greater capacity to cope with stress and recover from it more easily. Whether it's physical or emotional stress, our younger selves often had the energy and resources to "bounce back" from challenges without experiencing long–term effects.

However, as we age that natural resilience begins to decline. Our ability to recover from stress diminishes, and we might notice that events or traumas we once brushed off are now taking a toll. The truth is that the trauma or unresolved stress was always there, but when we were younger, our bodies could better manage it. As we grow older and our coping mechanisms weaken, the trauma we pushed aside starts to surface more prominently and now it demands our attention.

This is a common experience and aligns with a timeless principle in healing: trauma that is ignored or left unresolved doesn't simply disappear. If we don't deal with it sooner, it tends to resurface later in life. The stress and trauma that once seemed manageable in youth can start to weigh us down as we age and manifest in ways that can more profoundly affect our mental and physical health. This is why addressing trauma and stress early on, or at least when it begins to make itself known, is so important. Ignoring it only postpones the inevitable and can make it more difficult to deal with in the long run. The key is to recognize that healing is always possible, but the sooner we begin, the easier it is to regain control and find balance in our lives.

> **IMPORTANT NOTE:**
> When it comes to fight, flight or freeze mode, which you will be reading more about as you continue, it's important to understand which one is your dominant reaction. Personally, as a child, I would always go into *freeze* mode where I felt stuck and couldn't move. If I did something wrong or was scolded, I couldn't move. It was like my feet were cemented to the ground. As an adult, this happened a lot and became a big problem in relationships, jobs and daily life. I also had a little bit of *flight or flee* mode. Rarely did I have *fight* mode. Now, I've started to have a healthy level of fight mode response. The strategy for me was to recognize every time this happened and then use exercises to overcome the feeling and reactions. I would just recognize the freeze mode, *breathe* and *make* myself physically move. That was the first couple steps for me. From then on, it became easier and easier.

Knowing which one is dominant for you is very important, so going forward, take a moment to think of how you naturally respond to stressful situations. That way, you can strategize and employ techniques to overcome adversity.

Breaking Down PTSD

Post–Traumatic Stress Disorder ("PTSD") is a complex condition that can significantly impact someone's life. PTSD typically develops after experiencing or witnessing a traumatic event, such as combat, sexual assault, natural disasters, accidents, or other life–threatening situations. PTSD can manifest in various ways, including flashbacks, nightmares, intrusive thoughts, and intense physical and emotional reactions triggered by reminders of the traumatic event. These triggers may include sights, sounds, smells, or specific situations reminiscent of the trauma. Symptoms can start within 3 months of the traumatic event or even take years before you see any negative symptoms.

Western treatment for PTSD often involves a combination of psychotherapy, medication, and coping strategies. Cognitive–Behavioral Therapy ("CBT") is a common approach aimed at identifying and modifying negative thought patterns and behaviors related to the trauma. Exposure therapy, a type of CBT, gradually exposes individuals to traumatic memories or triggers in a safe environment to help them cope and reduce fear responses. Medications, (if you choose to go that route) such as selective serotonin reuptake inhibitors ("SSRIs") or serotonin norepinephrine reuptake inhibitors ("SNRIs") may also be prescribed to manage symptoms like depression, anxiety, and intrusive thoughts.

This book offers a wide–ranging toolkit of insights, knowledge, wisdom, practices, and techniques—blending both Western medical approaches, alternative medicine and Eastern wisdom—to support you and your life.

> **IMPORTANT NOTE:**
> Don't let the idea of medication scare you. However, you don't have to lean on medication as your only support! Do the work and use the techniques to identify and get to the root causes of disorders, such as those identified in this book. These techniques are excellent tools for anyone, regardless of whether they choose to go down

the route of medications. In addition to professional treatment, self–care techniques such as mindfulness, relaxation exercises, physical activity, and social support can play a crucial role in managing symptoms and promoting overall well–being.

PTSD is a complex and individualized condition, requiring patience, time, and ongoing support to effectively manage symptoms and work towards healing and recovery. Another way of looking at PTSD is by looking at how it exists in and for us. After experiencing something traumatic, our minds and bodies interpret the experience in a certain way to "define it." We then "upload" that information into our brain and limbic system. It's just like what happens when we download something and then upload it onto a computer's hard drive for storage and safekeeping. Why does this happen? It's so if we encounter another situation congruent with or mostly congruent with the initial traumatic experience, then our body will send a signal that there is danger. Our body then decides if we need to flee, fight or freeze.

So, a triggered response is a response from a past painful experience—the "past" or "post trauma." That's different than if you are having intrusive thoughts and bad vibes about a situation that you may be in at "the moment." This helps highlight some of the differences between fear and/or anxiety in the moment versus a fear response from a past trauma (the PTSD).

There is a similarity with how people respond to traumatic situations, but some just might interpret trauma more intensely than others. However, if someone is in a low/moderate state of stress for long enough they might start to store their situation as PTSD as well, i.e. staying in toxic relationships, work environments, etc.

Let's now delve a little deeper into the psyche. There are three layers of the psyche that relate to PTSD and anxiety. First, there is the subconscious where the PTSD gets stored. Second, there is the conscious mind where we have our everyday fears, doom scenarios, conscious thoughts, and overthinking. Third, we have what is in between the subconscious and conscious mind called "automatic thoughts."

Generally, automatic thoughts are the thoughts that seem to happen just under the radar of your conscious mind. In this case, they are usually about fears, self–doubt, and the doom and gloom that we all sometimes experience. Sometimes, if you can be aware enough you can catch yourself thinking them, we've all done it! We'll touch more on this in Chapter 7, Cognitive Behavior Therapy.

PTSD symptoms generally fall into four categories:

Intrusive Memories: You might experience unwelcome, distressing recollections of the trauma, flashbacks that make you feel as though the event is happening again, or nightmares about what occurred. Even reminders—people, places, or situations—can trigger intense emotional or physical reactions.

Avoidance: You may go out of your way to avoid thinking or talking about the event, and steer clear of people, places, or activities that bring the memory to mind.

Negative Changes in Thinking and Mood: Persistent negative beliefs about yourself, others, or the world can take hold, alongside ongoing feelings of fear, guilt, anger, or shame. You might struggle to recall important details of the trauma, feel emotionally numb or disconnected from loved ones, and lose interest in activities you once enjoyed.

Altered Physical and Emotional Reactions: Known as hyperarousal symptoms, these can include an exaggerated startle response, hypervigilance, irritability or angry outbursts, risky or self–destructive behavior, difficulty sleeping, and trouble concentrating. You may also notice physical signs of distress—sweating, rapid heartbeat, trembling—when faced with reminders of the trauma.

In young children (six and under), PTSD may present as repetitive play that reenacts aspects of the event or frightening dreams that don't always directly reference what happened.

Symptom intensity often fluctuates. Times of general stress or anniversaries of the trauma can provoke more severe reactions. Even everyday triggers—a car backfiring, a news report, a movie or music—can bring back vivid memories and feelings long after the original event. Recognizing these patterns is the first step toward seeking effective treatment and reclaiming your sense of safety and well-being.

What is C–PTSD?

C–PTSD is **Complex PTSD**, which is unfamiliar to many people. C–PTSD is caused by prolonged exposure to or chronic trauma. People with C–PTSD often experience the same or similar symptoms as PTSD. The difference comes from the type and length of time someone experiences trauma. Note that when I discuss PTSD, I also mean C-PTSD.

Most people experience at least one traumatic event during their lives, and about a quarter of those people go on to develop PTSD. No one really knows how many people have C–PTSD. Often, a person develops C–PTSD if they have prolonged stress, anxiety and/or panic or prolonged exposure to trauma. C–PTSD can develop after childhood trauma, bullying, traumatic or toxic relationships, being gas lit for long periods, assault and/or similar events. People that end up with C–PTSD also generally experience self–esteem issues, impulse control issues, shame and guilt, and/or feeling like they no longer have value.

Other Risk Factors for C–PTSD Can Include:
- Child trafficking
- War/being a prisoner of war
- Repeated assault/sexual assault
- Childhood abuse or neglect

- Prolonged domestic violence (including mental and emotional violence)
- Feeling trapped with no hope
- Repeatedly witnessing violence or abuse
- Multiple traumas

If this feels like a lot, I'm going to recap and put this all together in easy-to-understand scenario at the end of the chapter and again, we'll bring it all together in the last chapter. Let's keep learning about what's going on in that noggin of yours.

Limbic system: Your limbic system is the part of your brain that handles emotions, memory, and basic survival instincts. The limbic system is at the heart of panic, anxiety, and PTSD. Here are its four key players, in plain language.

Amygdala: Think of the amygdala as your fear center, the brain's alarm bell. It constantly scans for danger—real or imagined—and when it senses a threat, it lights up and sets off your fight-or-flight-or-freeze response. In PTSD, the amygdala is often "stuck on," triggering fear even long after the danger has passed.

Hippocampus: This little seahorse-shaped area files away memories and tags them with context: "where," "when," and "how." Your brain and hippocampus stores images, smells, sensations, sounds and anything else that seems necessary. Why does it do this? Because the brain and the mind need to understand the scary thing that happened, with the intention of avoiding that trigger and situation in the future.

In high stress, the hippocampus can get scrambled, so traumatic memories remain as raw emotional flashes rather than tidy past events. That's why a veteran might relive a combat scene at the sound of fireworks. The brain hears and sees the fireworks and goes, "Run, Alert!" In this book, we are going to guide you on how to rewire this. Just reading this and helping your logical thinking brain and mind understand this, is the first step.

Hypothalamus: Serving as your internal thermostat, the hypothalamus turns on stress hormones via the HPA axis and controls your heartbeat, breathing, and digestion. When the amygdala screams "danger," the hypothalamus responds by flooding your body with cortisol and adrenaline—perfect for running from a bear but exhausting when falsely triggered by anxiety.

Thalamus: Acting like a relay station, the thalamus directs incoming sensory information—sights, sounds, touch—to the amygdala, hippocampus, and higher brain centers for processing. In panic, it can become hyper–active, sending everything through the fear circuitry and escalating that "something's wrong!" feeling.

The brain in all its glory is constantly talking to each of its parts. When these four areas misfire—over–sensitive alarms in the amygdala, jumbled memories in the hippocampus, an overactive stress response from the hypothalamus, and a hyper–alert thalamus—they create the vicious loop of PTSD flashbacks, generalized anxiety, and sudden panic attacks. Learning how to calm this emotional network with breathing, grounding, therapy, and lifestyle tools is key to rewiring your brain's "fear wiring" for good.

Imagine your brain is like a security system: the AMYGDALA is the alarm bell, the HIPPOCAMPUS is the memory file cabinet, the HYPOTHALAMUS is the control panel that pumps out warning lights (stress hormones), and the THALAMUS is the switchboard that sends every noise and sight to those parts. If the alarm is too sensitive, the file cabinet gets messy, the control panel goes haywire, and the switchboard is on constant alert, you end up with a nonstop "threat detected" feeling.

Learning simple tools—like slowing your breath, grounding yourself in the moment, talking it out, and healthy habits—helps you reset and quiet down that overactive security system so it only goes off when there's real danger. Again, we'll go over this again a couple times while putting it all together in an easily digestible way.

The HPA Axis

The HPA axis is a collection and connection of structures that regulate the body's stress response, including the hypothalamus, pituitary gland and the adrenal glands. This is one of the systems of our endocrine system that is affected by PTSD and C–PTSD and many other functions and disorders. Prolonged PTSD can cause the HPA axis to dysfunction, which can create disharmony in the mind and body. In PTSD, the HPA axis systems talk to each other to release hormones. Let's see what a healthy HPA axis looks like:

When it's working properly, your HPA axis is like a smart power manager in your phone that keeps everything running smoothly:

1. **Daily energy boost**: It follows a regular schedule, gently raising cortisol each morning so you wake up alert and ready to go, then tapering it off toward evening so you can wind down and sleep.
2. **Quick response to real emergencies**: If you actually face danger—say, you narrowly avoid being hit by a car—your HPA axis kicks in to give you a burst of adrenaline and cortisol, so you react quickly and move out of harm's way.
3. **Balanced metabolism**: Those stress hormones help free up stored energy (glucose and fats) when you need it, whether that's for a workout or simply getting through a busy day.
4. **Immune regulation**: Cortisol helps dial down inflammation once a threat has passed, preventing your immune system from overreacting and causing chronic inflammation.
5. **Mood and memory support**: In normal amounts, cortisol helps consolidate everyday memories in your hippocampus and keeps your mood stable—too much or too little, and things start to go awry.

In short, a healthy HPA axis times and tailors its "power boosts" so you stay alert when needed, recover quickly afterward, and maintain balanced energy, immunity, and mood in your day–to–day life.

A person with PTSD can suffer from an insufficient amount of cortisol and then the person can't handle stress very well. Also, they can't RECOVER from a stressful event anymore. This is when people start to feel a "burnout." That's when you find yourself in a heightened state of stress and anxiety throughout the day and having trouble sleeping. When your parasympathetic system is overwhelmed, it's unable to restore your body to a state of calm and relaxation.

Symptoms of HPA Axis Dysfunction:
- Major depressive and anxiety disorders
- Memory problems
- Increased risk for cardiovascular problems
- Increased risk for diabetes, obesity, metabolic dysfunction immune system dysfunction (including autoimmunity disorders, increased cytokines—the proteins that help regulate the immune system, and chronic low-grade inflammation)
- Hormonal dysfunction – weight gain, low libido, blood sugar imbalances, thyroid issues
- Energy and sleep disturbances – tired but wired – fatigue
- Mood and mental health – anxiety, depression, brain fog, irritable and more

Before moving on, I want to share another way to look at PTSD from a Hebrew literature perspective: when exposed to a traumatic event, the emotional/psychological system is flooded with more stimuli than it can contain and process; the stimuli remain in the system in their raw, unprocessed state; and then occasionally return, forcing their way in to the person's awareness in their original form.

As a result, the sufferer re-experiences the traumatic situation, as if it were occurring all over again. Images, memories, noises, and odors that were part of the original traumatic experience return in an overwhelming manner that can feel like an assault. Since this intrusive, uncontrollable experience is in and of itself traumatic, victims try to avoid anything that might remind them of the traumatic event, creating a cycle of the intrusion and avoidance. This cycle is the heart of PTSD. All mammals and other species have this similar stress system.

PANIC TO POTENTIAL TOOL:
Whenever possible, find support. It's those who surround you and support you that make a huge difference in how initial trauma gets stored or not stored in someone's body and psyche. The more support you have during and after trauma plays a key role in whether you develop PTSD or not. Please understand, you need to do the work, no one is going to do it for you!

A quick way that may help you with anxiety or hypervigilance is to take a moment in your day to NOTICE the little successes and positive things that happen in your daily life. Stop, notice, smile and give yourself a mindful pat on the back. I would do this to help pull me out of my anxious state and still do it when I get overwhelmed. This can help the nervous system be calmer and more regulated as well. People tend to skip over their successes for many reasons. You will read why in Chapter 7. This is a small but mighty exercise. Let's move on for now, we'll come back and tie all this together with some examples.

Breaking Down the Nuts and Bolts of Anxiety

Anxiety is often seen as a fear of the future. For many, this rings true. Take a moment to reflect on whether this resonates with you. While it's a common emotion, anxiety can manifest differently for everyone.

At its core, anxiety is the body's response to fear. It's that feeling of apprehension or unease, typically triggered by a perceived threat or danger. In this discussion, we'll explore the causes behind these sensations, the triggers, and the experience of fear, as well as strategies to manage it.

First and foremost, it's important to understand that anxiety is a normal human experience. It affects everyone to some degree and serves an essential role in our survival. Anxiety can help sharpen our focus and make us more responsive to stress. This is why a healthy level of anxiety can enhance performance. However, for some, anxiety occurs more frequently or intensely, prompting the need for better understanding and support.

When anxiety becomes overwhelming and starts to disrupt daily life, it's crucial to take conscious steps to manage it. Without intervention, anxiety can escalate into panic and other challenges. This moves into the realm of "unnatural." Stress, in my experience and from the insights of others, tends to build up gradually over time if it's unaddressed. Knowing this helps us better understand stress and its impact.

In today's fast-paced world, stress can mount quickly, prompting some to seek immediate relief through medication. While taking a pill may offer immediate relief and prove sufficient in some cases, it's important to acknowledge that it's not always the sole solution. Chances are, you're reading this because your current coping mechanisms aren't cutting it anymore. Perhaps you're seeking deeper self-understanding, grappling with significant life challenges, and longing for relief. Whatever your reasons, I want you to know that you're not alone. I've been where you are and so have many others.

Here is what ex–CIA intel officer Andrew Bustamante says about fear and anxiety: "anxiety keeps you alive, attentive, focused and keeps you learning." He also goes on to explain that our brain has two hemispheres, the right emotional side and the left logical side. The right emotional side reacts much quicker and the left logical brain much slower. With fear in an untrained person, our emotions that are processed very quickly. This causes an instinctive reaction to fear. When fear happens, your logical brain is slowly processing how scared to be. You need to learn to slow down your emotional brain and speed up your logical brain. CBT helps with this by helping you stop and think logically and rationally. The goal is to essentially reject the emotional part first so you can get objectively process the scenario. This is called Socratic thinking/questioning.

Stress is an inevitable part of life, but when it becomes excessive, it can fuel anxiety and panic. I'm genuinely grateful that you're reading this and taking a step towards understanding and managing your struggles. When anxiety starts to overwhelm us, it's essential to intervene consciously. Otherwise, it can escalate into more intense anxiety and panic situations.

Other observations and suggestions about anxiety from Bustamante that I like include:
- **Heightened Awareness/Preparedness**: anxiety increases our awareness of potential threats and helps us prepare. It sharpens our senses and makes us more alert, which can be beneficial in both personal and professional settings.
- **Driving Personal Growth**: anxiety can push us out of our comfort zones, forcing us to confront our fears and grow stronger. It challenges us to develop coping strategies and resilience, ultimately leading to greater personal development.
- **Enhanced Problem–Solving Skills**: dealing with anxiety requires us to think critically and develop problem–solving skills. This can translate into better decision making and improved ability to handle stressful situations effectively.
- **Improved Performance**: in some cases, anxiety can enhance our performance by providing a boost of energy and focus. This is particularly true in high–stakes situations where being on edge can help us stay alert and perform at our best.

By reframing anxiety as a tool rather than a hindrance, Bustamante suggests that we can harness its energy to drive positive change and achieve our goals. I believe this is key in managing anxiety.

Former Navy SEAL and CIA officer Shawn Ryan offers practical, no-nonsense advice on his popular "The Shawn Ryan Show," for anyone who freezes up in social situations. First, always give yourself an easy exit: drive yourself, book your own hotel room, or choose venues where you can leave on a moment's notice. Second, come armed with confidence—whether that's through a quick power-posing routine in the car, listening to an energizing playlist, or simply reminding yourself of past wins before you walk in. Third, establish a "code word" with a trusted friend or partner; when you utter that word, they'll know it's time to help you make a graceful exit. Fourth, remember you don't have to carry the conversation—most people love talking about themselves, so simply ask open-ended questions and let them share. Fifth, keep your drinks light: skip the hard liquor (stick to wine or soda water) so you stay clear-headed and in control. Finally, don't underestimate professional support: a few sessions with a skilled therapist can give you tools to reframe your thoughts, build resilience, and turn socializing from a source of dread into an opportunity for connection.

Let's go over one more idea behind anxiety: resistance to either your thoughts and/or feelings. The more you want it to go away, the more it builds and the stronger it might feel. It becomes a habit for the anxiety signals to keep firing in the brain. You have to start retraining the brain and give it different signals. Retrain your amygdala to help it feel safe and give it a different experience.

If you fight and resist the anxiety, the amygdala reads this as dangerous and fires off more energy to "help." This comes down the statement that, in a way, "what you fear, you attract." You have to start telling your body, literally with words, "I'm safe, there is NO danger." When you can't care less about anxiety, it will start to go away. It has a lot to do with the resistance, not what's actually happening. There will be a lot of ways to start working with your brain and balance the nervous system within this book. Keep reading!

The Problem with Social Media

In the last 20 years social media has taken over our lives and our attention. It has brought with it many gifts and beautiful things. It has also brought us some new anxieties, especially in our youth and younger generations. Here are *15 Key Statistics on Social Media and Mental Health* identified by brightfuturesny.com:

1. 71% of people who use social media agree that it's important to take a break from it.
2. 45% of social media users feel overwhelmed by the amount of information shared on social media.
3. 24% of teenagers say social media has a mostly negative effect on their life.
4. 70% of teenagers check social media several times a day.
5. 59% of adults who use social media report that it has impacted their mental health.
6. 41% of women on social media report feeling pressure to present themselves in a certain way.
7. 63% of people on social media report being lonely.
8. 37% of people on social media report feeling FOMO (fear of missing out).
9. 63% of parents believe social media is harmful to their children's mental health.
10. 32% of teenagers report being cyberbullied.
11. 40% of people on social media report feeling anxious or depressed after using it.
12. 60% of people on social media report feeling like they *need* to take a break from it.
13. 70% of teenagers believe that social media platforms do not do enough to prevent cyberbullying.
14. 42% of people on social media report feeling more insecure about their appearance after using it.
15. 37% of people on social media report being negatively impacted by political discussions on social media.

Social media brings us positive things as well, including:
- Connecting with family and friends;
- Finding like–minded people and groups;
- Learning new things;
- Posting/sharing your own creative ideas through videos and posts;
- Easily accessing news and information; and

- Getting support from others.

But with the positive, there is the negative part of social media, including:
- **Having unrealistic views of others/lives and feeling inadequate as a result (one of the biggest issues);**
- Bullying, spreading rumors, and misinformation;
- Lacking real in-person contact and interaction; and
- Resulting distraction/addiction to social media.

I personally see social media almost as a "drug" and believe it should be used responsibly, especially for parents with children. There's a growing movement starting in 2025, where experts advise no social media for children under 15/16 years of age.

In today's fast-paced, ever-changing world, anxiety has become a common response to the instability of our socio-economic landscape. This might not affect you specifically, but it's definitely a big factor for people. Unlike past generations who often followed a predictable path—learning a trade, inheriting a family business, or staying with one company for decades—modern life is marked by constant change. Careers are shorter, job markets are more competitive, and the traditional sense of stability that once came from long-term employment has largely disappeared. Instead, we now live in a society that rewards speed, adaptability, and relentless opportunity-seeking, often at the cost of inner peace and mental well-being.

This creates constant pressure to "keep up," to stay relevant, re-skill, hustle, and adapt. While this culture of possibility may offer freedom and innovation, it can also lead to chronic uncertainty. The nervous system thrives on safety and predictability, yet many people today are living in a kind of low-level survival mode, unsure of how long their job will last, whether their career is secure, or if they're falling behind. The pressure to constantly reinvent oneself can quietly wear down resilience, leading to burnout, overwhelm, and anxiety.

The looming presence of artificial intelligence ("AI") only adds another layer of stress. With rapid advancements in AI technology, people across various industries are now questioning their future roles. Will their job still exist in five years? Will they be replaced by a machine or algorithm? Even if the threat is only perceived rather than immediately, the fear of being replaced or left behind creates a very real psychological burden.

Anxiety in this context is not irrational—it's the body and mind responding to a world that feels unpredictable and uncontrollable. The key is not to ignore this anxiety but to understand where it's coming from. Building emotional resilience, developing a flexible mindset, nurturing community, and cultivating inner safety through daily routines, mindfulness, and purpose–driven work can help create a stronger foundation. In a world that keeps changing, your sense of self and grounded-ness doesn't have to. You may not control the economy, technology, or societal shifts—but with the help of this book and hopefully other support around you, you can adapt and change with the times and be both healthy and successful!

Breaking down the Nuts and Bolts of Stress:

Stress is an inevitable aspect of life, an integral part of the human experience. While stress is a universal experience, the challenge arises when it becomes excessive and overwhelms our capacity to cope. This is what led to mental and physical breakdowns. Stress is a spectrum that ranges from manageable stress to the less desirable kind of stress. However, stress isn't inherently good or bad. The thing with stress comes down to our ability to navigate and recover from stress so we can return to a state of relaxation. This state of relaxation is getting us back into known parasympathetic mode, essential for rest and restoration. The parasympathetic nervous system is what helps our body relax and conserve energy.

Throughout any given day, our bodies and minds accumulate stress. It's a natural process and is often one that is more easily managed in our youth where resilience tends to be more pronounced.

However, as we age, maintaining this resilience becomes increasingly challenging, particularly if we neglect our physical well-being.

As we get older and perhaps become less physically fit, our capacity to cope with, recover from, and alleviate stress diminishes. Techniques for stress management are instrumental in addressing this phenomenon. It's crucial to recognize that stress can manifest physically, often concentrating in specific areas like the neck, shoulders, abdomen, and lower back.

In subsequent chapters, we'll delve into strategies aimed at equipping you with tools to effectively manage stressful situations. Together, we will foster not just coping mechanisms, but genuine healing and empowerment. The ultimate objective is to facilitate a state of contentment, vitality, and abundance, which we all inherently deserve. The methodologies presented in this book are designed to facilitate stress management, recovery, and the restoration of our body's innate ability to contend with daily stressors effectively.

Shifting focus for a moment, I want you to think about some of the most common (but unhealthy) coping mechanisms for stress. Some people resort to alcohol, cigarettes, or other substances, while others may turn to behaviors like overworking, overeating, or engaging in addictive patterns such as excessive sex. If you find yourself relying on these substances or behaviors to navigate through life's challenges, know that you're not alone and that you can change these patterns.

You've come here with purpose. There exist alternative approaches that, if chosen, I firmly believe can offer you significant relief.

IMPORTANT NOTE:
Stress and anxiety place a significant demand on the body's resources, often causing it to burn through nutrients, vitamins, and minerals at a much faster rate. Over time, this can lead to real nutritional deficiencies, something many people don't realize. There's a

persistent myth that in the Western world, it's impossible to be nutrient deficient because we have easy access to food. But that simply isn't true. We live in a society where we are often overfed but undernourished. This important topic will be explored further in Chapter 3.

A Birds Eye View of Fear

Let's take a moment to talk about one of the most essential yet somewhat misunderstood emotions: fear, which some say stands for **F**orget **E**verything **A**nd **R**un. This may be a good tactic if you're in real danger or if it's your default setting, but let's look into it further.

Like all emotions, fear is experienced differently by each person. For some, it sharpens focus and even boosts performance under pressure—much like anxiety can. For others, it's paralyzing, taking over both the body and the mind.

At its core, fear is a completely natural biological response to either real or perceived threats. It sets off a chain reaction in your brain and body designed to protect you—a survival mechanism that helped keep our ancestors alive. But here's the question that really matters for us today: *What happens when fear goes too far? When fear stops protecting you and starts limiting your life?*

We did go over some patho–physiology earlier, but you don't need to understand all the science just yet, or at all if that's not what interests you. I'll be revisiting some of these ideas in later chapters, so you can absorb them at your own pace. For now, think of this section as a bird's eye view to get you started.

The Three Fear Responses: Fight, Flight, and Freeze

When your nervous system senses danger—whether real or imagined—it usually reacts in one of three ways: fight, flight, or freeze.

Fight means facing the danger head–on. Your body surges with adrenaline. Muscles tense. Your heart rate rises. In day–to–day life, this might show up as sudden anger, defensiveness, or trying to take control of a stressful situation.

Flight is about escaping. You may feel jittery, anxious, or panicked. You might physically want to run, or mentally disconnect by avoiding situations, people, or emotions.

Freeze happens when your system shuts down because neither fight nor flight feel possible. You may feel numb, stuck, or dissociated. Your body might feel like it's shutting down while your mind races—like slamming the gas and brake at the same time. You may even feel unable to move physically. This was me as a child. As an adult I often found myself in similar situations.

For many people with PTSD (like me), freeze becomes the default setting. It's not something we choose, it's our body doing what it thinks will protect us. But over time, staying in this state can make us feel like we're stuck in survival mode, unable to move forward. For years, my nervous system was locked in this loop. What started as unprocessed childhood trauma eventually spiraled into complex PTSD, chronic illness, autoimmune problems, and complete emotional and physical exhaustion. I couldn't work, maintain relationships, or even go outside without symptoms. I wasn't living, I was just surviving. Barely. That's why this book exists. To offer not just information, but practical tools to help you understand what's happening in your body and mind—and to remind you that healing *is* possible.

Today, I live a life I once thought was out of reach. I'm married, I'm thriving, and most importantly, I'm free from the daily grip of panic, PTSD symptoms, and chronic anxiety. I still have challenges—everyone does—but I'm no longer imprisoned by fear. That's what I want for you, too.

When someone with PTSD encounters a trigger, the body launches into survival mode. First, the sympathetic nervous system kicks in—the "fight or flight" system. Adrenaline and norepinephrine flood your system, increasing heart rate, raising blood pressure, and shutting down digestion. The body is gearing up to fight or run.

But when escape or confrontation isn't possible—especially if that was the case during past trauma—your system may switch to the freeze response. This is where it gets complicated. The parasympathetic nervous system, specifically through the vagus nerve, activates as well, causing the body to shut down. Now you're receiving both signals at once: act and shut down. This internal tug–of–war can feel like being frozen in place while your mind is spinning.

At the same time, your HPA axis—another key part of the stress response—is releasing cortisol, the main stress hormone. Cortisol helps you survive short–term danger, but when it stays elevated for too long, it leads to serious health problems like fatigue, anxiety, poor digestion, and even immune dysfunction.

Freeze, Dissociation, and Why You're Not "Crazy"

During freeze, the body may release natural opioids (like endorphins), which create a numbing or dissociative effect. It's like your body is giving you an "emotional painkiller" so you can survive the moment. You might feel foggy, disconnected from your surroundings—or from yourself. That's your brain doing its job, even if it doesn't feel great.

Your amygdala—the brain's fear center—gets louder, while your prefrontal cortex—the rational, thinking part of your brain—goes quiet. You can't think clearly or talk your way out of it because your system is trying to keep you alive, not have a philosophical discussion.

Once the danger feels over (even if it was just in your head), your nervous system tries to bring things back to baseline. But if this cycle repeats often—and remains unresolved—it becomes trauma, anxiety, panic, and chronic illness.

Why Understanding This Matters

None of these reactions mean you're broken. They mean you're human. These are survival systems that just got stuck in overdrive.

The more we understand what's happening inside us, the more we can move toward compassion, healing, and freedom. Tools like CBT, mindfulness, grounding practices and other exercises you'll learn in later chapters can help you work through these states and retrain your system toward safety.

This chapter is only the beginning. You don't have to know everything right now. The important thing is that you're here, reading, learning, and opening to a new possibility: that your body and mind are capable of healing and that fear, while powerful, doesn't get to run the show forever.

Innate Fears

From the moment we're born, our nervous systems carry built-in alarms for particular dangers. These innate fears require no prior experience to emerge:

- Fear of Falling: Infants placed on a visual cliff hesitate or cry, signaling a built-in caution against heights.
- Acoustic Startle: A sudden, loud noise triggers an involuntary flinch and distress—nature's way of alerting us to immediate threat.

Why it matters: These reflexive responses kept our ancestors from life-threatening falls and unseen predators, ensuring survival long before we had the luxury of rational thought.

Biologically Prepared Fears

Beyond what we're born fearing, our brains are primed to learn fear more readily for historically dangerous stimuli. These biologically prepared fears aren't present at birth, but require far less exposure to develop. For example:

- Snakes and Spiders: even without a bad encounter, most people can spot and react to these creatures faster than, say, a flower or a butterfly.
- Dangerous Heights: while babies must learn to navigate stairs, we're evolutionarily tuned to sense drops as hazardous.

Preparedness Theory: Psychology research suggests our ancestors who quickly learned to fear venomous animals or treacherous terrain were more likely to survive—and pass on those wiring patterns to us.

How These Fears Take Hold

Instinct vs. Learning: innate fears spring up fully formed; prepared fears emerge through minimal learning or by observing others' reactions.

Resistance to Extinction: Once lodged in our brains, prepared fears prove stubborn. Classical conditioning with a spider or snake can leave a lingering phobia if not carefully unlearned.

Innate fears are reflexive, present from birth, and critical for immediate survival. Biologically prepared fears require little exposure to learning, reflecting the threats our species faced over millennia. Preparedness theory bridges biology and psychology by explaining why certain fears "stick" so easily and persist so strongly.

By recognizing which fears are wired in us and which are learned, we gain powerful insight into our own reactions. These learned fears can function as a signal to identify what to work on. We can recondition ourselves so that these learned fears no longer inhibit us.

A Birds Eye View of Depression

We'll be diving deeper into this subject in later chapters, but for now I just wanted to give you a quick understanding and how it fits within the scope of this book.

Depression from a clinical perspective can offer valuable insight into its complexity. Depression is a multifaceted mood disorder characterized by persistent feelings of sadness, hopelessness, and a loss of interest in activities that once brought joy. Clinically, it's typically diagnosed when these symptoms last for at least two weeks and are accompanied by changes in sleep, appetite, and energy levels.

Those affected may struggle with concentration, experience feelings of guilt or worthlessness, and in more severe cases, have thoughts of self–harm or suicide. Depression impacts both mental and physical health, disrupting daily functioning, relationships, work, and overall quality of life. Its causes are varied and may involve a combination of genetic, biological, environmental, and psychological factors. Thankfully, effective tools from this book, including therapy and lifestyle changes, can help manage and alleviate symptoms.

Sometimes, not always, depression can feel like a heavy fog that refuses to lift. But just like clouds in the sky, these feelings can and do pass. It's easy to forget that during hard moments. Maybe you had a rough night of sleep. Maybe you argued with a loved one or had a difficult day at work. Perhaps something is brewing beneath the surface—something you haven't even named yet—but it builds and builds until it feels like a dark cloud hanging over you. Sometimes, that cloud just needs time to pass. Other times, it needs your attention. That's what this book is here for: to help you know the difference and to remind you that no emotional state is permanent. So please, keep going—and keep coming back to the tools that guide you home to yourself.

Research has revealed a strong link between depression, anxiety, PTSD and physical pain. This overlap is one reason why antidepressants are frequently prescribed for anxiety-related conditions as well. Both Eastern and Western healing systems offer valuable perspectives when it comes to addressing depression. In this book, we'll examine how depression can be interwoven with anxiety, panic disorder, adrenal exhaustion, and chronic fatigue. Understanding the scientific, emotional, energetic, and social dimensions of depression allows for a more holistic and compassionate approach to healing.

From a philosophical and existential standpoint, depression often stems from a lack of meaning, motivation, or personal growth. This can manifest as a willingness to settle for mediocrity or doing just enough to get by. When a person lives without clear goals, dreams, or a sense of purpose, especially one that extends beyond the self and involves contribution to others, it can drain their vitality and spark feelings of emptiness or disconnection. In Chapter 7, we'll explore how modern psychological patterns, when combined with a lack of structure or meaning, can contribute to emotional stagnation, stress, and depression.

Living a life with no focus on self, or one overly consumed by self-focus, can create a misalignment that feeds depressive states. Finding the balance between purposeful action and internal awareness is often a key part of restoring emotional health.

Human beings are naturally creative and expressive. We thrive when we're growing, building, and creating something meaningful. Without these outlets, we can start to feel stagnant, as though something essential is missing. While some people may find deep contentment in a simpler, more detached way of life—and that can absolutely be fulfilling—for many of us, a prolonged absence of challenge, growth, or self-expression can lead to a state of merely existing rather than truly living. Striking a balance between contentment and progress, between being and becoming, is often a key part of living a more purposeful and fulfilling life.

On an energetic or spiritual level, this mirrors some of the deeper psychological and energetic roots of depression. In Eastern philosophy, depression is often viewed as an imbalance between Yin and yang energies. it is typically associated with an excess of yin—feminine aspect, receptive, passive, cooling energy—without enough yang—masculine aspect, which brings action, drive, and movement. This perspective helps explain why states of stagnation, fatigue, lack of sunlight and emotional heaviness are so central to depressive experiences. We'll explore this more deeply in the chapters on yoga and qigong, which offer practical ways to restore this energetic balance through movement, breath, and awareness. Even when it comes to nutrition, the B vitamins are drivers of energy production at the foundation, which is a yang aspect.

Nutrition also plays a vital role in mental health and depression. We'll dive into this further in Chapter 3, but it's important to note here that malnutrition is far more common in the modern Western world than many people realize. Diets high in ultra processed and even moderately processed foods leave the body depleted of essential nutrients, contributing to inflammation, hormonal imbalance, and poor brain function. Shockingly, one in three adults is now estimated to have a metabolic disorder—a condition that's closely linked to both physical and mental health issues, including depression.

Here's a short list of common conditions linked to metabolic dysfunction: insulin resistance, fatty liver disease, diabetes, heart disease, hypertension, cancer, dementia, and more. These issues are often interconnected and can have a profound impact on both physical and mental health.

Even something as simple as gaining a clearer understanding of what panic and anxiety are—both physiologically and psychologically—can be incredibly calming in itself. This foundational knowledge will become especially useful later in the section on Cognitive Behavioral Strategies, where we'll explore how thoughts and perceptions directly influence the nervous system and our emotional responses.

Something that ties closely to depression is loneliness. Loneliness has significant negative impacts on both physical and mental health, including an increased risk of heart disease, stroke, cognitive decline, depression, anxiety, and even premature death. It can also weaken the immune system and raise the risk of certain chronic conditions. These kinds of effects are easy to overlook, which is why true health and well-being must be approached as a whole lifestyle—not just a diet or a quick fix. Some are even calling it a loneliness epidemic, as the numbers continue to rise. So, what can you do? It is incredibly important to build and sustain a community of friends and family. And I don't say that lightly. I personally used to shut people out of my life and avoid social situations, as I struggled with social anxiety myself. But I want you to know that the information and tools in this book can help. I am no longer socially anxious, and you don't have to be either (if that's something you struggle with). You'll find more techniques and insights in later chapters. I can tell you with full confidence that working on trauma and anxiety makes a huge difference when it comes to connecting with others.

Depression is more than just "feeling sad." It's a complex biological state in which several body systems become unbalanced. At its core, depression often involves dysregulation of the brain's monoamine neurotransmitters (serotonin, norepinephrine, and dopamine), which help regulate mood, motivation, and pleasure. When their levels or receptor sensitivity drop, the brain's reward circuits and emotional centers (like the prefrontal cortex and limbic system) struggle to function properly.

Meanwhile, the HPA (hypothalamic–pituitary–adrenal) axis—our central stress response system—can get stuck "on," flooding the body with cortisol. Chronically elevated cortisol disrupts sleep, impairs immune function, and can even shrink the hippocampus, the region responsible for learning, memory, and contextualizing emotions. Elevated inflammatory markers (like cytokines) often accompany this process, further interfering with neurotransmitter production and receptor activity.

Together, these chemical and hormonal shifts create a feedback loop of low energy, poor sleep, impaired concentration, and persistent negative thinking. Over time, that loop deepens, making even small tasks feel overwhelming. Understanding depression's pathophysiology reminds us that it's a medical condition—not a character flaw—and that addressing neurotransmitters, stress hormones, inflammation, and neural health all play a part in finding relief and restoring balance. This is why and how depression fits into everything we're talking about in this book.

Is Anxiety Genetic?

In my experience, I believe it can be—at least to a degree. My mother struggled with anxiety and panic disorder, and I believe that influenced my own tendency toward anxiety. Interestingly, my older brother did not develop anxiety in the same way. I suspect that certain early–life factors made me more susceptible. I've learned that my mother was very anxious during my birth, and as an infant, I was often held while she was experiencing high anxiety and panic situations herself. There was also more tension and conflict between my parents during my early years compared to when my brother was a baby.

Looking back, I believe it was a combination of these early experiences, my natural temperament and constitution, and my environment that set the stage for anxiety. I grew up shy, introverted, and sensitive, which made me more prone to absorbing and internalizing the anxiety and turmoil around me. In tense situations, I would feel immediate guilt and freeze—my body storing those moments as trauma. Over time, my HPA axis encoded these experiences as patterns of fear, contributing to PTSD and a life marked by chronic fear and dissociation.

Research suggests that roughly 30% of anxiety may be tied to genetic factors. I believe it may be less than 30% but still can be a factor. For me, it was a blend of inherent tendencies, learned behaviors, and the lack of a strong parental model to guide me through fear. Without that guidance, I couldn't outgrow those early patterns on my own.

If you're struggling with persistent anxiety, this book is here to offer support and guidance. I know how difficult it can feel when those feelings won't pass, leaving you feeling hopeless, helpless, or worthless. I used to feel that way, too. I isolated myself, avoided social events. I often turned around halfway to gatherings or declined invitations from friends. But I no longer live that way, and you don't either. Change is possible. I can tell you that from my own experience.

My journey toward transformation involved extensive personal healing, therapy, and deep introspection. Along the way, I've come to understand my natural introverted tendencies, while also realizing that I can be outgoing and confident, especially when sharing something I'm enthusiastic about or when in an entertaining role. This self-awareness has been invaluable, especially when navigating social interactions, something that can feel challenging for those of us who've experienced anxiety or trauma.

That said, past traumas left me with deep insecurities and a persistent sense of vulnerability, making it hard to feel safe around others. Recognizing this was a major turning point for me. I've come to see that working on yourself is essential before entering into new relationships. While some people may view this as an excuse, I see it as an important and necessary step. On the other hand, while continuing to do personal work is crucial, finding the right person for you can also greatly support your healing. That's been the case for me. My wife is my biggest supporter and an immense source of encouragement. Just having someone who truly understands you and offers consistent support is incredibly healing. If I hadn't done the inner work—studying CBT, reflecting on my past, and gaining clarity—my relationship might have been far more challenging. We've talked about this openly. While there's no way to know exactly how things would have turned out otherwise, we both agree that the work we did beforehand made all the difference.

When dealing with PTSD or the lingering effects of trauma, it often feels like pieces of your true self are slipping away. Trauma builds emotional walls and survival patterns that make it hard to access who you really are. You may find yourself reacting from a place of fear or self–protection, rather than from a place of genuine expression. This can blur the line between your true self and the coping mechanisms you've developed just to survive.

Many people go through life without ever fully exploring or understanding themselves. They may not feel the need to question their habits, motivations, or reactions—and that's perfectly okay. Everyone is on their own journey. But for those who feel the pull to reconnect with their true self, the healing process—while challenging—can be deeply rewarding. Rediscovering who you are beyond old wounds allows you to build a life aligned with your values, strengths, and authentic desires. Each step toward self-awareness brings you closer to a more fulfilling existence, free from the patterns of the past.

We are social creatures by nature. It's simply how we're wired. While there are always exceptions, most of us eventually crave connection because it is part of our natural state of being. Some people are naturally more social, while others are less so. That's simply the beautiful spectrum of human experience.

IMPORTANT NOTE:
Your natural state is *not* one of anxiety.

If you're living with constant stress, panic, feelings of unworthiness, hopelessness, or irrational fear, something happened to put you in this state—likely through a combination of experiences over time. This book is here to help uncover what those experiences may have been and provide tools to change the patterns they created. Your natural self is not defined by perpetual tension, physical pain, or fear of human connection.

Many people, however, have never had the chance to develop the healthy discernment needed to connect with others who genuinely align with them. This often affects romantic relationships. It's one reason we see so many people caught in "toxic" or abusive relationships or why cycles of abuse repeat across generations, as parents unconsciously pass down unhealed pain to their children. This phenomenon, called *trauma bonding*, occurs when someone forms a deep attachment to a person who causes them harm, often through a cycle of abuse followed by moments of positive reinforcement.

I've experienced my own share of abusive relationships. And while the path to healing was long and often difficult, I gradually broke free. Today, I am happily married to my wife, and we share a fulfilling life together. I now have the time, energy, and peace of mind to sit here and write this book—a guide I hope will help others transform their lives and rediscover their own natural state of calm, confidence, and connection. This is what's called the *Hero's Journey*. People have written fables about it for thousands of years.

This section is crucial, so let's emphasize it again: **throughout your life, certain experiences may have been registered by your body and brain as trauma—experiences that mask your true, genuine, and beautiful self**. It's important to understand that the only time you were truly helpless was as a baby. As an adult, you now have the power to take action, sift through the emotional baggage, and reveal your authentic self.

When we carry unresolved trauma or PTSD, our natural tendency is often to dissociate, to disconnect from our bodies. This happens because our bodies become places of remembered pain, and we instinctively try to distance ourselves mentally, emotionally, and energetically from that. Some people turn to substances like drugs, alcohol, or sugar as coping mechanisms to avoid these feelings. This book provides insights and techniques to help you heal stuck trauma, process it, and either integrate or release it (often a combination of both) so you can live fully present within yourself once again.

Another issue we spoke about earlier is social media. Comparing ourselves to others is a significant challenge in today's world. Social media, while an incredible tool for connection and entertainment, can easily become another drug if not used wisely, especially for young people. It can foster unhealthy comparisons. As parents and mentors, it's vital that we help children navigate it with awareness, guidance, and support.

These comparisons happen subtly. It's easy to forget that most people don't look or live the way they present online. We may find ourselves subconsciously comparing our real lives to curated images and feeling pressured to be something we're not. This comparison trap isn't limited to women either; men compare themselves to other men's lives, bodies, careers, and success as well. Even while writing this book, I caught myself feeling unworthy when I looked at all the "competition" out there. This tendency affects us all—it's human nature. The key is to stay mindful of it, build resilience with discipline and self-awareness, and not allow it to undermine our sense of worth or purpose.

This section highlights the importance of understanding trauma, recognizing our worth, and learning to stay grounded within ourselves, instead of allowing comparison or disconnection to define us. Through mindful practices and conscious awareness, you can reconnect with your true self and nurture your unique path forward.

Now, emotionally speaking, I want you to read this part slowly. Our own emotions, especially those rooted in fear and trauma, create a cycle that leads to depression. Negative emotions such as fear, anger, guilt, or shame, often tied to past traumas, can become powerful forces when left unprocessed. When fear and PTSD responses remain active, they trigger our body's stress response repeatedly, releasing hormones like cortisol and adrenaline. Over time, this creates a state of constant vigilance and anxiety. This "fight-or-flight" state drains us emotionally and physically, leaving little room for relaxation, joy, or even peace.

The impact of these emotions also extends into how we see ourselves and others. Trauma often brings feelings of guilt or shame, where we blame ourselves for things that were never our fault. These feelings can lead us to believe we are unworthy or that we somehow deserve the pain we're feeling—further isolating us from the people and support we need. Over time, this isolation can reinforce the idea that we are alone in our struggles, compounding feelings of sadness and hopelessness.

Living under the weight of fear or trauma also creates **patterns of avoidance.** We begin to avoid situations, people, or memories that might trigger painful responses. This keeps us from experiencing life fully and leads to a sense of detachment and numbness. The more we avoid, the more disconnected we feel from ourselves and others. Over time, this detachment can lead to apathy. Eventually, this emptiness can set the stage for depression, a state where emotions feel dulled, life loses its meaning, and a sense of despair can take hold.

Understanding this cycle is essential if we want to break free from it. By addressing and processing these deep-seated emotions with self-compassion—and with professional support if needed—we can begin to let go of the weight of fear and trauma. This allows us to reconnect with our natural state of well-being and rediscover purpose, joy, and a deeper connection to ourselves and to life. This cycle of trauma can feel like an endless loop, but let's break it down simply. A traumatic event creates a negative charge in the mind and body. We then try to avoid it because it's painful, this leads to feelings of dissociation and apathy. For some, our natural drive for balance kicks in, others, maybe not so much, but instead of bringing relief, it brings feelings of shame, guilt, worthlessness, or other negative emotions. And so, the cycle continues.

This is why therapists and teachers often emphasize the need to confront fears and trauma—gently and skillfully. That is the purpose of this book: to guide you in a way that makes examining your trauma feel less overwhelming. While it's not a replacement for a personal coach or therapist, it offers a framework to help you face your pain with greater courage and clarity.

Godspeed.

Takeaways from Chapter 2

- This program is adjunctive. It can be used alongside any other healing modalities or approaches you are currently practicing in your life. The goal is to complement and support your existing efforts, not to replace them.
- Nutrition as you'll see in the next chapter, plays a crucial role in pain, panic, anxiety, depression, and stress—especially considering the harmful additives and nutrient–depleting effects of modern processed foods. The quality of what you eat has a direct impact on how your nervous system and brain function.
- Learning the patho–physiology of PTSD, Trauma and anxiety can be an important step in your recovery.
- Another key point to remember is that we don't have to be in the situation to feel the fear. When your brain senses danger, whether real or perceived, it releases catecholamines—including adrenaline—and triggers the fight–or–flight response. This flood of neurotransmitters can create feelings of panic, anxiety, fear, nervousness, and worry, even when there is no actual threat present.
- It's also important to understand that sustained stress and anxiety can have a detrimental effect on the body's immune system. Chronic stress can either suppress immunity or cause it to become dysregulated, sometimes contributing to autoimmune conditions, where the body mistakenly begins to attack its own tissues and systems—leading to dysfunction across multiple areas of health.
- A small component of anxiety can have a genetic origin—but this should not be used as an excuse. Knowing this may offer some insight, but the true work begins by examining your own life and beginning the healing process. It's worth having conversations with your parents or caregivers to uncover any childhood experiences that may have contributed to PTSD or trauma you are carrying today.

- Panic, in its simplest form, is your body going into full fight–or–flight mode when it's not supposed to. It is an extreme overreaction by your system—interpreting a non–threatening situation as if it were a serious danger.
- Anxiety itself is normal—we all experience it. It's that nervousness you feel before giving a speech or taking an exam. But when anxiety becomes overwhelming and unmanageable, that's when it needs to be addressed—before it progresses to panic.
- Stress is also normal. Everyone experiences it. There's good stress, such as the natural stress your body experiences during a workout or the boost you get right before an important performance. The real problem is not whether stress is "good" or "bad"—it's whether you have the ability to recover from it. The inability to recover, combined with too great an amount of stress at one time, is what wears down the system. Many people cope with stress by turning to substances—alcohol, recreational drugs, or unhealthy behaviors. But there are healthier ways to regulate stress, and this book offers many natural tools you can turn to instead.
- Finally, it is vital to remind yourself: you are not wrong, broken, or backward. You are amazing. You might simply need a little support in certain areas—and everyone does! Depression can feel like a dark cloud overhead, but it is often temporary. We all have bad days, bad weeks, or even longer funks that feel hard to shake. In Chapter 3, you'll learn how much of a role nutrition plays in depression—and how making changes in this area can make a profound difference in how you feel.
- I hope you'll stick with me through to the very last chapter - 11, also the CBT chapter 7, where I bring everything we've covered together into clear, easy-to-digest steps designed to inspire real, lasting change.

Chapter 3
Nutrition and Supplementation:

"Let food be thy medicine and medicine be thy food."
— *Hippocrates*
"The greatest wealth is health."
— *Virgil*
"Take care of your body. It's the only place you have to live."
— *Jim Rohn*

Now, more than ever, nutrition is critical to overall health and well–being. Much of what I'll share in this section may challenge some of the beliefs you've grown up with. There are many myths and misconceptions around health and nutrition that have been passed down over generations. At the end of this book, you'll find a curated list of trusted resources—Western doctors, cardiologists, nutrition experts, functional medicine, Eastern medicine practitioners, and others—who may help guide you even further.

From a young age, I've always had a knack for looking beneath the surface and uncovering the root causes of issues. Over the years, I've come to realize something very clear: while people today are often overfed, they are also severely undernourished. In other words, we do not have a calorie problem, we have a nutrition problem. Nutrient insufficiency is widespread in modern society—especially here in the West—largely due to the overconsumption of processed and ultra–processed foods. These foods often lack the essential vitamins, minerals, and micronutrients that the body requires to thrive.

On top of this, many processed foods are filled with compounds known as anti–nutrients that can interfere with nutrient absorption and digestion, and in many people, can contribute to harm and dysfunction in the body (not everyone, but certainly to varying degrees.) Unfortunately, many supplements on the market also fall short of providing what the body truly needs in bioavailable and absorbable forms.

This section of the book shares my personal journey, research, and the practical insights that have helped me—and countless others—achieve better health through nutrition. My hope is that this inspires you to question conventional wisdom and begin developing your own deeper understanding of nutrition and how it can transform your well-being.

IMPORTANT NOTE:
This section is for information purposes only. I am not a doctor. I am not prescribing, diagnosing, or recommending anything specific. I am simply sharing what has helped me personally, along with information that I encourage you to explore and research on your own, especially when it comes to nutrition and supplementation.

I am not affiliated with any company or individual mentioned in this book. I receive zero kickbacks or any other compensation for mentioning any person, product, or brand here.

Now, let's dive into supplementation, popular healthy diets, a few fun facts about nutrients, and some of the most common undiagnosed nutritional disorders affecting people today.

Basic Foundational Supplements:

Magnesium

The queen of them all. This is such an important mineral that I want to spend a little extra time on it. Personally, I use many different types and brands of magnesium. I also use electrolyte powder which comes with some magnesium. Magnesium is a big one because it's involved in over 300 biochemical reactions in the body. It plays a vital role in regulating muscle and nerve function, blood sugar levels, blood pressure, and in the creation of protein, bone, and DNA.

Unfortunately, our food supply, especially our soil, is now deficient in magnesium, which only amplifies the problem we face in modern diets. That's why supplementation is often necessary. And this is with actual whole foods; it's even worse with ultra–processed foods, which typically contain little to no magnesium at all. This is yet another example of being overfed but undernourished.

You may wonder why you can't just get a blood test to check your magnesium levels. The truth is that we can't accurately measure magnesium or certain other electrolytes this way. Only about 1% of magnesium in the body is found outside the cells in blood or plasma—this is what's tested. But the other 99% is stored in bones and muscle tissue, where standard blood tests can't detect it. We really don't know what those cellular levels are.

Here's what happens: the body is designed to keep your blood pH and electrolyte levels as stable as possible for survival. So, if magnesium levels drop, your body will start pulling magnesium from bones and muscles to maintain proper blood levels. That's why blood tests almost always show magnesium as "normal," even when your tissues may be depleted. Unless you are severely deficient or are dealing with serious chronic disease, your blood levels can appear fine while your body is running on empty behind the scenes.

Another factor that worsens magnesium depletion is a high sugar or high carbohydrate diet. The more sugar you consume, the more magnesium is required to process it—and this can quickly deplete your stores. This is why low magnesium is often correlated with insulin resistance, diabetes, and a range of metabolic disorders.

Vitamin D3 – K2

Most people today are not getting nearly enough Vitamin D either from the sun or from supplements. In fact, Vitamin D deficiency is one of the most overlooked yet critical pieces of the puzzle when it comes to healing from chronic illness, autoimmune issues, PTSD, and supporting overall nervous system resilience. Based on my research, Vitamin D levels should be at least 50 ng/mL or higher—and optimally around 70 ng/mL or even more. If your test result shows 30 ng/mL or below, you are likely deficient—even though many lab ranges will falsely reassure you by showing "green" at 30. This is simply outdated and does not reflect what the body truly needs for optimal immune and nervous system function.

In my own lifestyle, I make it a priority to get natural sunlight first thing in the morning. This does two things: first, it helps set and regulate my circadian rhythm, which is crucial for sleep, mood, and hormonal balance. Second, it allows my body to naturally begin producing Vitamin D through the skin. Since I am lighter–skinned, I aim for about 20 minutes a day in the sun when possible—arms, legs, and face exposed.

But here's the truth: for most people, sunlight alone isn't enough year–round, especially if you live in northern climates, spend lots of time indoors, or wear sunscreen frequently (which blocks Vitamin D synthesis). That's where supplementation comes in.

If you do supplement—and I highly recommend looking into it—Vitamin D3 (cholecalciferol), not D2, is often better. More importantly, I strongly recommend that Vitamin D3 always be paired with Vitamin K2. Why? Because Vitamin D helps your body absorb calcium, but Vitamin K2 helps direct that calcium to the right places (bones and teeth) and prevents it from depositing in soft tissues like arteries. This is vital for long–term cardiovascular health. The ratio you want is roughly 10:1 Vitamin D3 to K2, and most good supplements already have this balance built in.

Personally, I take about 5,000 to 10,000 IU of Vitamin D3 per day. Once you're there, you may not need as much daily for maintenance, depending on your sun exposure and individual needs.

IMPORTANT NOTE:
If you're not getting enough Magnesium, it will be difficult or unable to get Vitamin D levels high enough, on top of, if you have a high carb, processed food diet and lifestyle.

If you have autoimmune conditions, pay close attention here: Vitamin D is absolutely essential. One of the key drivers behind immune system dysregulation—and even autoimmune expression—is Vitamin D deficiency. Your immune system simply cannot function properly without sufficient Vitamin D. This is even more critical if you are dealing with chronic illness or nervous system dysregulation. Low Vitamin D creates an uphill battle that no amount of other healing practices can fully overcome until it is corrected. Sometime Doctors will prescribe high doses of Vitamin D once a week. This is not natural and tends not to work long term. Your body likes to have daily or consistent intake for longer term healing and health.

If I could give one simple, affordable biohack that offers a massive return on investment for almost everyone, it would be: optimize your Vitamin D3 and Vitamin K2 intake and pair it with daily sunlight and movement.

Nitric Oxide

This is something that many people don't hear much about when it comes to healing from chronic illness, PTSD, anxiety, or even supporting cardiovascular and brain health, but it can be a true game-changer.

A personal example: my wife struggled with long COVID for well over a year. She had shortness of breath, developed asthma, was using an inhaler almost daily, needed regular breathing treatments, and experienced itchiness in her chest/ lungs, fatigue, brain fog, and a host of other frustrating symptoms. We tried nearly everything: supplements, red light therapy, energy work, Chinese medicine, Pilates, but her body was too depleted to tolerate much, and nothing was bringing real relief.

That's when I came across Nitric Oxide research. We learned how essential it is for blood vessel dilation, oxygen delivery, and overall cellular health. I immediately got her on a high–quality Nitric Oxide supplement, and the results were nothing short of remarkable. Within a couple of days, her breathing improved dramatically. The shortness of breath was gone, her energy levels returned, and she was able to work normally again—something we hadn't seen in months. For her, it was a huge missing key.

I only recommend Nitric Oxide products developed by Dr. Nathan Bryan. I've spent hours listening to his lectures, reading about the decades of research, and learning how much effort (and millions of dollars) has gone into creating effective, clinically validated Nitric Oxide products. There's a lot of junk on the market, so I urge you to be selective—this is one supplement where quality and formulation matter greatly.

But here's the exciting part: you can also support your body's natural production of Nitric Oxide through biohacking and nutrition— no fancy pills required (though supplements can help when needed).

Here are some ways to naturally boost Nitric Oxide:
- **Sunlight**: spending time in natural sunlight stimulates Nitric Oxide production in your skin. Another reason to get outside first thing in the morning.
- **Movement**: exercise, especially aerobic movement (walking, cycling, running) boosts Nitric Oxide naturally by increasing blood flow and stimulating the endothelial lining of blood vessels.
- **Nose breathing**: breathing through your nose increases Nitric Oxide production in the nasal passages, which helps with

oxygenation and circulation. This is one reason I emphasize diaphragmatic breathing in this book.
- **Red and near–infrared light therapy**: this stimulates Nitric Oxide release in cells and enhances mitochondrial function. Another great biohack.
- **Nutrition**: certain foods (only if you can tolerate these) are rich in Nitrate, which is converted to Nitric Oxide in the body:
    - Beets and beetroot juice
    - Arugula
    - Spinach
    - Swiss chard
    - Cilantro
    - Lettuce
    - Celery
    - Dark chocolate (high cacao content)
    - Pomegranate
    - Watermelon (contains L–Citrulline, which supports Nitric Oxide)

You'll notice a pattern here—real, whole foods and a natural lifestyle support this essential molecule.

Why is this important in the context of PTSD, anxiety, and chronic illness? Because Nitric Oxide improves blood flow, oxygenation, and cellular energy (mitochondrial function). It also has a role in reducing inflammation and helping the body shift from sympathetic fight–or–flight dominance into a more balanced state. It supports neuroplasticity, immune function, and even helps with vagal tone—a big part of healing the nervous system.

For my wife, it was a night–and–day change. And in my own healing journey, I now see Nitric Oxide as one of the most overlooked tools for people struggling with fatigue, breathlessness, brain fog, cardiovascular issues, or lingering symptoms post–infection or trauma.

As with anything in this book, I encourage you to do your own research, and if this resonates, explore adding more natural Nitric

Oxide support into your lifestyle. Usually, you can increase this as you change your lifestyle and diet. The results can be remarkable.

Electrolyte powder

This is something I use daily as part of my healthy lifestyle and maintenance routine. Personally, I use Dr. Eric Berg's Electrolyte Powder, though there are other good brands out there if you choose wisely.

Electrolytes are absolutely essential for basic life functions—they help maintain electrical neutrality in your cells and are critical for generating and conducting electrical impulses in your nerves and muscles. Without proper electrolyte balance, your entire system becomes unstable—especially when you are healing from chronic illness, PTSD, anxiety, or autoimmune conditions where the nervous system is already under significant stress.

The key electrolytes your body needs include sodium, potassium, chloride, magnesium, calcium, phosphate, and bicarbonates. These minerals are crucial for proper hydration, muscle function, nerve signaling, heart rhythm, and even mental clarity.

Here's something most people overlook: if you are drinking lots of water and your urine is consistently clear (or if you're exercising, sweating, or in hot environments) you are naturally losing electrolytes at an increased rate. While hydration is critical, it can dilute your electrolyte levels if you don't replenish them. Ideally, urine should be a light yellow color throughout the day. If it's always completely clear, you may be flushing out more than just toxins—you could also be losing precious minerals.

Once you reach your mid–thirties or older—or if you are showing signs of electrolyte deficiency—it becomes wise to consider adding electrolyte support into your daily routine. This is particularly true for anyone with chronic stress, burnout, adrenal fatigue, or PTSD, as these conditions can dramatically impact electrolyte balance through prolonged stress responses and hormonal imbalances.

Common symptoms of electrolyte deficiency include but are not limited to:
- Muscle–related issues: cramps, spasms, twitches, weakness, or numbness
- Digestive issues: constipation, diarrhea, or abdominal cramping
- Mental issues: confusion, irritability, anxiety, or lethargy
- Heart–related issues: irregular or rapid heartbeat, palpitations, or arrhythmia
- Other common symptoms: dizziness, lightheadedness, headaches, or frequent urination

In the world of biohacking, electrolytes are a foundational tool for anyone pursuing optimal performance, nervous system resilience, and mitochondrial health. Without proper electrolyte balance, the electrical systems of your body can't function efficiently. This can amplify feelings of anxiety, worsen fatigue, and impair mental clarity, which is why I consider electrolytes to be a key pillar of any holistic healing program.

IMPORTANT NOTE:
When selecting an electrolyte powder, avoid those loaded with sugar, artificial sweeteners, or junk additives. A clean, high–quality formula—like the one I use—is worth investing in.

Remember, small daily habits like adding electrolytes can create profound shifts in your overall sense of vitality, energy, and emotional stability. As always, listen to your body—and adjust as needed.

Cod Liver Oil

I personally use either Dr. Berg's Cod Liver Oil capsules or a liquid cod liver oil from a high–quality source, such as Life's Fortune Pure Icelandic Cod Liver Oil. Cod liver oil is one of the most nutrient-dense supplements you can take. It provides nearly your full daily value of Vitamin A, Vitamin E, and Omega–3 fatty acids—with the added bonus of a small amount of Vitamin D as well. Because this is an animal–based product, the vitamins and nutrients are delivered in their most bioavailable form, meaning your body can easily absorb and utilize them. I highly recommend cod liver oil over any plant–based Omega–3 or Vitamin A supplement. If you are dealing with chronic illness, nervous system dysregulation, or immune challenges, this is one of the few supplements that provides foundational support for cellular repair, brain health, and anti–inflammatory balance.

Omega–3

Omega–3 fatty acids are critical for both mental health and physical resilience. They support brain function, reduce inflammation, and help regulate mood, making them incredibly helpful for those recovering from PTSD, anxiety, and chronic illness. While plant–based Omega–3s (such as flaxseed or chia) can provide some benefit, the conversion rate to the usable forms—EPA and DHA—is very low. That's why I always recommend getting your Omega–3s from a marine source, such as fish oil or cod liver oil. In today's world, most people have a poor Omega–3 to Omega–6 ratio due to the heavy use of seed oils in processed foods. Correcting this ratio through supplementation can make a noticeable difference in inflammation levels, brain clarity, and emotional balance. Omega–3s are also powerful support for heart health, joint health, and even gut lining repair, making them a must - have in any comprehensive healing program.

B Vitamins

B vitamins play a critical and often overlooked role in both mental and physical health. I've found them to be an essential part of my healing process and one of the most profound tools in recovering from PTSD, anxiety, chronic fatigue, and brain fog. Modern life depletes our B vitamins rapidly—through stress, processed–food diets, alcohol, sugar, and even certain medications. Supplementation can make a world of difference when done properly.

Vitamin B1 (Thiamine) is, in my opinion, one of the most important and most undervalued B vitamins—especially in today's world. Thiamine is absolutely vital for brain function and mental clarity. It plays a key role in energy production, helping convert food into fuel and supporting overall brain metabolism. Low B1 can leave you feeling mentally sluggish and physically fatigued. Thiamine also supports nerve signaling, helping improve mood regulation and reducing anxiety. It enhances cognitive function, supporting memory and focus, and it plays a major role in how your body responds to stress, by nourishing the adrenal glands. Importantly, Thiamine provides neuroprotection, shielding your brain cells from damage and supporting long-term mental resilience.

Personally, I take both Thiamine HCL and Benfotiamine. I follow the guidance of Elliot Overton, whose work on this topic you can find on YouTube. This combination, along with flush Niacin (Vitamin B3), has been absolutely life-changing for me. And yes, I say that seriously—these simple vitamins had more impact on my health and healing than many expensive interventions I've tried.

Vitamin B3 (Niacin) is another powerhouse. I highly recommend the flush version—nicotinic acid—as it provides much higher benefits than the non-flush form. The niacin "flush," a warming sensation caused by blood vessel dilation, actually supports circulation and detoxification—two things the chronically ill and anxious body desperately needs. Niacin supports the production of key neurotransmitters, including serotonin and dopamine, which help regulate mood and combat depression. The enhanced circulation from the flush effect improves mental clarity and brain function, while its anti-inflammatory properties target underlying inflammation that can contribute to anxiety and depression. Niacin also supports energy production at the cellular level and aids in detoxification, which is crucial if you're dealing with a toxic burden from stress, trauma, or chronic illness. Start slowly, as the flush can be intense. If needed, niacinamide offers some of these benefits without the flush, though it is not as potent in my experience.

Vitamin B6 is another essential player. However, it is important to be cautious: too much B6 over an extended period can potentially cause nerve issues in sensitive individuals. I personally cannot supplement B6, so I take my B vitamins separately, not in a pre-blended B-complex. Many people, however, are deficient in B6, especially if they experience anxiety, mood swings, or hormonal imbalance. You can ask your doctor to check your levels through a simple blood test.

Methylfolate (B9) is a highly bioavailable form of folate—much preferred over synthetic folic acid. If you have an MTHFR gene mutation (which is more common than you'd think), your body may not process standard folic acid efficiently. Methylfolate bypasses this issue, allowing your body to use it effectively. Gary Brecka, a human biologist I respect greatly, speaks about the critical importance of Methylfolate for mental health, DNA repair, and detoxification, especially in those dealing with chronic stress or genetic vulnerabilities.

Methylcobalamin (B12) is another vitamin I consider foundational for mental and physical healing. Always choose Methylcobalamin, not cyanocobalamin, as it is the bioavailable form your body actually uses. B12 plays many crucial roles: it helps convert food into energy, reducing the fatigue so common in depression and chronic illness. It supports the production of neurotransmitters like serotonin and dopamine, enhancing mood and helping regulate emotional stability.

B12 also promotes nerve health, improving brain function and mental clarity. It supports memory, focus, and overall cognitive function—key for anyone struggling with brain fog or trauma-related mental fatigue. Additionally, B12 is essential for red blood cell production, helping deliver oxygen throughout the body and supporting sharper mental alertness.

The takeaway? B vitamins, when understood and used wisely, can be a game-changer for anyone working to heal from PTSD, anxiety, chronic fatigue, or depression. In the modern world, with our stress-heavy lifestyles and depleted food supply, supplementation of these key vitamins is often not optional—it is essential.

Here's the kicker: naturally in humans, we are supposed to be getting most of our B vitamins and some other nutrients from our gut microbes. We'll talk about these here soon, but they produce B vitamins for us in our GUT, and we absorb those!

Iodine

Iodine is one of the most overlooked yet essential minerals for human health. I personally take about 3–4 drops of Lugol's 2% solution daily, which gives me roughly 6–8 mg of a blend of iodine and potassium iodide. I consider it one of the "super supplements," right up there with magnesium and thiamine.

Unfortunately, iodine has gained an undeserved bad reputation—largely due to confusion dating back to the 1950s, when researchers used radioactive iodine in mouse studies. This led many to associate *all* iodine with toxicity. But here's the truth: natural iodine is not radioactive. It's essential for life. The fear that followed those studies is irrational and misplaced, yet it still lingers in our culture today.

Every cell in your body needs iodine, but it's especially vital for the thyroid gland, breast tissue, prostate, ovaries, and other hormone-regulating organs. It plays a central role in metabolism, energy regulation, immune health, and even cognitive function. And yet, despite its importance, it's estimated that 95–97% of people in Western countries are deficient—often without realizing it.

Why are so many people low in iodine?

First, our food system. Most people aren't eating iodine-rich whole foods anymore. Instead, they're eating processed or ultra–processed products stripped of minerals. Add to that the fact that modern agricultural soils, especially in areas like the Great Lakes region, are severely depleted of iodine, and the deficiency becomes nearly unavoidable.

Second, we're bombarded daily by halogen elements like fluoride, chlorine, and bromine, which compete with iodine in the body and often displace it at the cellular level. These substances block iodine absorption and wreak havoc on our endocrine system.

You'll find bromine in more places than you'd expect: it's used as a flame retardant in electronics, clothing (especially synthetics), insulation, furniture foam, carpets, and even car seats. It's also found in pesticides (like methyl bromide), certain pharmaceuticals, hot tub and pool disinfectants, plastic products, dyes, inks, and even some hair and skincare products. It's even found in our food, specifically processed foods, including baked goods and beverages. Fluoride and chlorine are common in municipal tap water and dental products. When these halogens build up in the body, they occupy iodine receptor sites in the thyroid and other tissues, disrupting hormonal balance and cellular function.

So, what can you do?

Start by reintroducing iodine into your system—both through iodine–rich foods like seaweed, shellfish, fish eggs, and pastured eggs, and through supplementation. (Think of the traditional Japanese diet, which contains some of the highest iodine levels in the world.) Contrary to popular belief, iodized table salt isn't reliable, it loses its iodine quickly once exposed to air and contains only trace amounts to begin with. It's just enough to prevent goiters, but not nearly enough to support optimal health.

The iodine I recommend is Lugol's solution. If you're new to iodine, start with the 2% version. You may also come across a stronger 5% version—just start with fewer drops. Dr. David Brownstein is one of the most well-respected voices on iodine today, and I encourage you to check out his work if you want to go deeper into the science and protocols.

One thing to be aware of: when you begin supplementing with iodine, it will start displacing fluoride, bromine, and chlorine from your tissues. This can trigger a detox response, sometimes called a Herxheimer reaction. These "healing symptoms" might include fatigue, headaches, skin breakouts, stomach upset, fatigue, or mood swings—not because iodine is harming you, but because your body is eliminating stored toxins. That's why it's wise to start slow, go steady, and support your detox pathways (e.g., with magnesium, selenium, hydration, and rest).

Iodine is foundational. If you've been struggling with chronic fatigue, brain fog, hormonal imbalances, thyroid issues, or even low-grade depression or anxiety, this may be one of the key missing pieces. And in a world full of environmental toxins, it's more important than ever to reclaim this ancient mineral and restore your body's natural balance.

Essential Co-Factors to Support Iodine Supplementation (*also beneficial for overall wellness, detox, and chronic health support*)

When beginning iodine supplementation—especially Lugol's iodine—it's critical to ensure your body has the necessary co-factors to use it properly and safely. These nutrients not only support iodine's beneficial effects but also help your body detoxify the halogens (bromine, fluoride, and chlorine) it displaces. Many of these co-factors are also excellent foundational supplements for anyone looking to improve their energy, mental clarity, and immune resilience. Such co-factors include:

Zinc

Zinc plays a crucial role in hormone production, including thyroid hormones, and supports a stable immune response. It functions complement iodine, which is essential for the synthesis of thyroid hormones, which influences overall metabolic and immune health.

Selenium

This is a *key* co–factor for iodine, especially in supporting thyroid hormone production and protecting the thyroid during detox. Most supplements provide 100–300 mcg per serving, which is within the safe range. Brazil nuts are nature's richest source—just 1 to 2 large nuts per day is plenty.

> **IMPORTANT NOTE:**
> Don't take Brazil nuts *and* a selenium supplement at the same time—choose one or the other to avoid excess.

B–Complex Vitamins

This includes B1 (Thiamine), B2 (Riboflavin), B3 (Niacin or Niacinamide), B5, B6, B7 (Biotin), B9 (Methylfolate), and B12 (Methylcobalamin). I personally avoid B6 because I'm sensitive to it—too much can cause neuropathy–like symptoms (such as tingling in the legs at night). While this reaction is relatively rare, it's something to be aware of. A blood test confirmed my sensitivity, so now I use a B–complex without B6.

Magnesium + Electrolytes

Magnesium supports detox, calms the nervous system, and is involved in over 600 enzymatic reactions. I take around 300–400 mg per day from food and supplements.

- I use Dr. Berg's Electrolyte Powder, which contains magnesium citrate, and add magnesium glycinate for a gentler, more

calming effect.
- Be aware that too much citrate can cause a laxative effect—listen to your body.

Vitamin C

Vitamin C is essential for adrenal health, immune support, and neutralizing oxidative stress during detox.
- A dose of 500–1000 mg per day is ideal for most people.
- If you're symptomatic, avoid sugary fruits and juices. A little raw honey is okay now and then, especially if eaten with probiotic-rich foods like yogurt.
- On a carnivore or low-carb diet, your vitamin C needs may be lower due to less oxidative stress and glucose competition.
- Fermented foods like kimchi and sauerkraut are great natural sources if tolerated.

PANIC TO POTENTIAL TIP:
Start with half the recommended dose of supplements and increase slowly over 1–2 weeks. Many people are deficient in these vital nutrients and don't realize the impact that restoring them can have on mood, energy, and detoxification.

Guidance for Sensitive Individuals or Chronic Illness

If you have chronic symptoms, autoimmune conditions, or have never experienced a detox or Herxheimer reaction before, proceed with care. The detox process from halogen displacement (bromine, fluoride, chlorine) can trigger healing symptoms—fatigue, skin breakouts, stomach upset, brain fog, mood shifts, etc. It's not the iodine itself, but what it's *dislodging*. This is where co-factors play a vital role.

Start Low, Go Slow

If you're new to iodine or sensitive, start with just *half a drop* of Lugol's 2%. You can do this by adding 1 drop to a small glass of water and drinking half. Stay at this level for a week or two before increasing.

- 1 drop of Lugol's 2% provides approximately 2.5–3 mg of iodine/iodide.
- Many experts recommend building up to 12.5–25 mg/day, but this depends on your individual needs and detox capacity.

Final Thoughts

Dr. David Brownstein is one of the most respected voices on iodine therapy. His decades of work, research, and clinical experience have helped thousands reclaim their thyroid and hormonal health. I encourage you to watch his lectures or read his material. If possible, work with a functional medicine practitioner or naturopath familiar with iodine therapy.

The bottom line: iodine is *incredibly* powerful, but it requires the right support. With the proper co–factors and patience, it can become one of the most transformative additions to your wellness journey.

Organic food

Organic foods are especially valuable because they typically contain little to no glyphosate—a widely used herbicide found in weed killers. Glyphosate has been shown to negatively impact the gut microbiome by harming beneficial bacteria, which can lead to digestive issues and increase the risk of chronic health conditions. This is one of the many reasons to choose organic whenever possible.

Equally important is minimizing processed and ultra–processed foods. These are often high in added sugars, unhealthy fats, preservatives, and artificial ingredients. While they may be calorie-dense, they're typically nutrient–poor, which can lead to both overconsumption and malnutrition. Ultra–processed foods also tend to be low in fiber and essential nutrients, making it easy to eat more while still depriving the body of what it truly needs to function and heal.

Another hidden challenge to nutrient absorption comes from anti-nutrients—natural compounds found in many plant-based foods that can interfere with how our bodies absorb and use nutrients. Common anti-nutrients include:

- **Oxalates**, found in foods like spinach, beets, and almonds, which can bind to calcium and may contribute to kidney stones in susceptible individuals.
- **Phytates**, present in grains, legumes, and seeds, which can reduce the absorption of zinc, iron, and other key minerals.
- **Gluten**, which in sensitive individuals, can cause inflammation and digestive issues, especially for those with celiac disease or gluten intolerance.

While some people tolerate anti-nutrients without noticeable problems, others—especially those with chronic inflammation or digestive issues—may need to be more cautious. If you're already dealing with chronic illness or poor gut health, reducing plant-based foods high in anti-nutrients and processed grains may be especially beneficial, grains especially. (See the research of Dr. William Davis and Dr. Natasha Campbell McBride).

Conditions like insulin resistance and fatty liver disease can further impair how your body absorbs and uses nutrients. For instance, insulin resistance affects glucose metabolism and often leads to systemic inflammation and low energy. When combined with a poor diet, this can spiral into a cycle of malnutrition and metabolic dysfunction.

Note that not everyone reacts the same way. One person might handle oxalates just fine, while someone else might be dealing with fatigue, pain, or digestive distress because their system is overloaded. The average person can tolerate about 200–300 mg of oxalates per day, but if you're at risk for kidney stones, that number drops to around 100 mg or less. These are things many doctors and experts don't always talk about but should, especially for those of us with chronic health issues.

Excess sugar and food additives, especially artificial sweeteners, are strongly linked to anxiety, depression, and metabolic disorders. On top of that, one of the biggest and most overlooked problems is low stomach acid. Your stomach needs sufficient hydrochloric acid to properly break down proteins and absorb minerals. Without it, you may experience bloating, nutrient deficiencies, and chronic fatigue—even if you're eating the right foods.

Most people, even many of the experts I've followed, don't talk enough about this underlying cause: a significant number of digestive issues like GERD, acid reflux, and even bloating or indigestion often stem not from "too much stomach acid," but from a dysregulated vagus nerve and low vagal tone. The vagus nerve, which plays a central role in the parasympathetic nervous system, is responsible for regulating many involuntary functions, including digestion. One of its key roles is controlling the esophageal sphincter—the valve that should remain tightly closed to prevent stomach acid from flowing upward.

When someone is under chronic stress, dealing with PTSD, burnout, anxiety, or insomnia, the vagus nerve can become dysfunctional. In this state of dysregulation, it may fail to properly signal the esophageal sphincter, allowing acid to rise into the esophagus, creating symptoms like heartburn, tightness in the chest, or even the feeling of a lump in the throat. In other words, the problem often isn't "too much acid," it's the body's inability to control where that acid goes.

One nutrient often overlooked in this conversation is Vitamin B1 (Thiamine). A deficiency in B1 can significantly impair vagus nerve function and contribute to autonomic nervous system imbalance, including symptoms like poor digestion, acid reflux, fatigue, dizziness, and even panic. Thiamine is essential for energy metabolism in the nervous system, and when it's depleted—often due to chronic stress, a high-carbohydrate diet, alcohol, or nutrient-poor processed foods—the vagus nerve can't perform optimally.

Supporting the vagus nerve through proper nutrition (including Thiamine), deep breathing, cold exposure, gentle vagus nerve massage, and mindfulness practices can help restore balance to the parasympathetic system and improve digestion from the root. Instead of suppressing symptoms with acid blockers or antacids, we must ask: why is the body failing to regulate its own systems—and how can we support it in healing? Healing the nervous system isn't just about calming the mind; it's also about restoring foundational functions of the body, one of which is healthy digestion.

Lastly, there are several other underlying disorders that can directly contribute to your symptoms. I won't go into detail here, because each one could be a book in itself. I encourage you to take this as an invitation to research and explore what might be going on in your own body and use that knowledge to fuel your healing journey.

Reducing processed foods, choosing organic when possible, and being mindful of anti-nutrients is a powerful step toward better digestion, stronger immunity, and improved energy.

Histamine Intolerance and Sensitivity

Histamine is a naturally occurring biogenic amine that functions as both a neurotransmitter and an immune mediator in the body. It plays a crucial role in several physiological processes, including immune response, inflammation, and neurotransmission. During infections or inflammation, histamine is released to signal other parts of the body to respond to the threat and promote healing.

However, under conditions of chronic stress or dysbiosis (an imbalance in the gut microbiome), the lining of the gut can become compromised. This can impair the body's ability to regulate histamine properly. As a result, individuals may become overwhelmed by the histamine present in both foods and the environment. When the gut lining is damaged, the production of diamine oxidase (DAO), an enzyme responsible for breaking down histamine, is reduced. This can lead to a buildup of histamine in the body, triggering a range of uncomfortable symptoms, such as headaches, digestive issues, skin rashes, and other signs of histamine intolerance. If histamine is not properly broken down, these symptoms can become chronic and severely impact quality of life. Do some research on DAO enzymes including histamine issues of course. I've to a few hours of Histamine and DAO lectures and it can be very important information if you are dealing with Histamine like so many people are.

Histamine Intolerance happens first in the body and then the worsening effects become MCAS, which can have even worse symptoms, we'll go into that next. Sometimes it's not about 100% eliminating histamine foods and drink, which is almost impossible, but to better work on the body and strengthen the digestion to handle the natural histamine. It's like when we talk about strengthening the body to handle natural stress better.

This is an important area as it has a lot to do with health issues such as autoimmune disorders and more, which can contribute to mental health, mood concerns and anxieties. There are so many people with this in modern times because of toxins in the food, water, air and environment!

Toxins are a huge part of the Histamine issue. Household items, endocrine disrupting items like lotions, soaps, shampoos, cleaning liquids, creams, detergents, perfumes, Febreze's, carpets, all plastics of any kind we come into contact with such as Phthalates, PFAS, PVC, BPA, and more. You need to start getting all natural products, please do some research and find the products that work for you! My wife likes the app Yuka to research products.

Fatty liver will also contribute to histamine intolerance and MCAS. The liver can't process histamine properly and you might need what's called SAM–e supplement as well. I have not taken this supplement. Please do your research on this and talk to your doctor. Sam–e (in my research) has helped people with histamine/ MCAS symptoms and more.

Other than that, look into what foods are giving you symptoms and limit or take them away for a period of time, but you will need to take some time and talk to a medical professional or do your own research to get onto a protocol that works for you. Functional medicine can be a good place to start. There's more on what to do but this will give you some knowledge and get you ahead of the game.

MCAS

Mast Cell Activation Syndrome (MCAS) is a condition in which the body's mast cells—special immune cells that help mediate allergic responses—become overly sensitive and release excess amounts of chemical mediators like histamine. Unlike a classic allergic reaction, MCAS is not typically immediate or tied to one specific allergen. Instead, it can be a chronic or recurring condition that mimics allergies but often comes without obvious cause. This hypersensitivity can lead to a wide array of symptoms such as hives, itching, sinus congestion, mucus buildup, rashes, and inflammation. For many people, these symptoms are triggered after eating, especially meals that are rich in histamine or include ingredients that provoke mast cell responses. Fermented foods, aged cheeses, alcohol, smoked meats, and certain leftovers are common culprits.

In my own journey, MCAS symptoms showed up as extreme food sensitivities. Nearly every meal caused some reaction, which added a new layer of stress to eating. Unlike typical food allergies, MCAS tends to present a broader, more generalized immune activation, making it difficult to pinpoint a single trigger. Managing it involves supporting the immune system, reducing histamine load, calming inflammation, and identifying food and environmental triggers.

Postural Orthostatic Tachycardia Syndrome (POTS)

POTS is another condition I came to understand firsthand. POTS occurs when your heart rate increases significantly—more than 30 beats per minute—upon standing from a seated or lying position. This isn't just a random quirk; it's your body struggling to regulate blood flow and nervous system responses. For me, even walking up the stairs or rising from the couch would cause lightheadedness, a racing heart, or a crash in energy levels. It often overlaps with other nervous system dysregulations, which leads us to the next point.

Dysautonomia

Dysautonomia is a broad term for dysfunction of the autonomic nervous system, the part of your body that controls automatic functions like heart rate, breathing, digestion, and body temperature. It's a key player in PTSD, panic, anxiety, and many chronic illnesses. Dysautonomia is often the result of prolonged stress, trauma, fear, or emotional overload. Your body gets stuck in fight–or–flight and loses its ability to return to rest–and–digest. This can lead to symptoms like irregular heart rate, blood pressure swings, digestive issues, cold hands and feet, sleep disturbances, and more. One major breakthrough in my own healing came from learning about Vitamin B1 (Thiamine). After studying the work of Elliot Overton and others, I realized how critical Thiamine is for nervous system health. I wish I had started sooner. It's especially important if you're dealing with fatigue, anxiety, or autonomic dysfunction.

One strange but telling symptom I had was an inability to sweat normally. Sometimes I'd overheat with no sweat at all; other times I'd sweat excessively in random situations. PTSD would trigger adrenaline surges that kicked off my POTS symptoms, threw off digestion, and worsened my MCAS flare–ups. It was a domino effect—and dysautonomia sat at the center.

Chronic Inflammation (including from autoimmunity, and infections) is a silent contributor to so many issues, including weight gain, pain, autoimmune diseases, diabetes, hormonal imbalances, and even mitochondrial dysfunction. Sometimes inflammation is driven by low–level infections or immune dysfunction that never fully resolves. Symptoms like chronic fatigue, brain fog, recurring aches, and "flu–like" malaise can be signs your body is fighting off something below the surface.

Fat–Soluble Toxins

Fat–soluble toxins are some of the hardest to remove from the body. Unlike water–soluble toxins that pass through urine, these compounds get stored in fat tissue, the brain, and organs like the liver. This includes persistent organic pollutants (POPs) like dioxins, PCBs, and organochlorine pesticides; heavy metals such as mercury and lead; industrial chemicals like BPA and phthalates; solvents like benzene and xylene; and even certain medications. These substances lodge deep in the body and can disrupt hormones, mood, immune function, and brain health. Mold toxins, known as mycotoxins, also fall into this category and are notoriously difficult to detox without proper support.

Unfortunately, the body can't just pee these toxins out. They rely on healthy liver function (especially phase I and II detox pathways), proper bile production, and regular elimination. If you're constipated, not sweating, eating poorly, or having sluggish bile flow, these toxins may recirculate and continue wreaking havoc. Supporting natural detox pathways through movement, clean nutrition, binders (like charcoal or chlorella), sweating, and stress reduction can help your body slowly release these stored toxins. It's not about a quick fix—it's about giving your body what it needs to cleanse and repair over time.

Healing from these complex layers—MCAS, dysautonomia, POTS, inflammation, and toxin buildup—requires a gentle, methodical approach. But healing is possible. These conditions are deeply interconnected, and the body has a powerful ability to reset when given the right support.

Different "Diets" and Ways of Eating

The following is compiled from my own personal experience and from doctors and other experts who have been extremely helpful in my studies and research in a healthy lifestyle, particularly different ways of eating and "diets."

IMPORTANT NOTE:
Please don't begin doing any extreme dieting without researching and studying yourself OR having a professional guide you. Rule of thumb, always talk to your doctor, medical professional or nutritional expert before going into any dieting, fasting or shifts in your eating habits. This is just a rough guide to show you what's out there and again, what has helped me in having a healthier lifestyle.

Personally, right now I eat an animal–based diet, with a combination of ketogenic and carnivore diet. Low carb and as low inflammation as possible as well.

Low Carb Diets – Low Inflammation Diets:

Consider a healthy ketogenic diet coupled with intermittent fasting. Let's do a mini deep dive into this one. Ketogenic diet has been around since the 1920's and the military has been researching keto for a good reason.

A healthy ketogenic diet combined with intermittent fasting (IF) can be a powerful approach to improving metabolic health, supporting weight loss, and enhancing overall wellness. Here's a breakdown of each component and the benefits they provide together:

A Healthy Ketogenic Diet

A ketogenic diet is high in *healthy* fats, moderate in protein, and very low in carbohydrates. By drastically reducing carbs, the body shifts from using glucose as its primary fuel source to burning fats, producing ketones for energy. Key components of a healthy ketogenic diet include:
- Healthy fats from avocados, olive oil, coconut oil, nuts, seeds, and fatty fish.
- Prioritizing high–quality protein sources like grassfed meats, eggs, and organic poultry.

- Low Carbohydrates focusing on non–starchy vegetables like leafy greens), while eliminating sugars, grains, and high carb foods.

Everyone needs to find out which carbs they can tolerate or not. I personally react to pretty much all rice and sometimes corn and wheat/glutens. I tolerate a bowl of oatmeal as a small afternoon meal sometimes, but not at night. For dinner, I usually eat grassfed beef or organic chicken, often with organic sour cream or plain thick homemade yogurt. If I eat grains, it's usually quinoa with grassfed/organic butter (when I can find it) and salt.

IMPORTANT NOTE:
Eat protein first and then whatever carbs you may be eating. This cuts down on the glucose spike. Adding cinnamon especially with things like oatmeal really help curb the glucose/insulin spike. This is extremely important for anyone diabetic or pre–diabetic and insulin resistant people (most people). You DON'T want to be insulin resistant. You WANT to be insulin sensitive.

What is Intermittent Fasting?

Intermittent fasting is an eating pattern that cycles between periods of eating and fasting. During fasting periods, the body uses stored energy, which can aid in fat burning, cellular repair, and hormone regulation. When combined, a ketogenic diet and intermittent fasting can offer synergistic benefits.

There are several fasting methods, but popular ones include:
- 16:8: fasting for 16 hours and eating during an 8–hour window—this is the common starting point.
- 18:6 or 20:4: extended fasting windows for a shorter eating period.
- 5:2 day method: eating normally for five days and significantly reducing calorie intake for two days.

I've personally only used the 16:8 method so do your research and look into what works best for you. If you try things like this just transition slowly and try it for short durations.

With low-carb, high-fat intake, the ketogenic diet reduces blood sugar spikes and crashes, which can lead to improved blood sugar control and insulin sensitivity, so your blood sugar is more stabilized. Adding IF to this regimen can lower fasting blood sugar levels and help stabilize glucose throughout the day.

Enhanced Fat Burning and Weight Loss

Ketosis: the ketogenic diet naturally induces ketosis, where the body uses fat for fuel. Intermittent fasting can accelerate this state by depleting glycogen stores and forcing the body to tap into fat reserves faster.

Increased lipolysis: intermittent fasting further enhances fat breakdown (lipolysis), helping the body become more efficient at burning stored fat for energy.

MCT Oil: Medium-chain triglyceride (MCT) oil is a powerful addition to any diet, especially if you're seeking clean, sustained energy. Unlike long-chain fats that require a more complex digestive process, MCTs are rapidly absorbed through the small intestine and transported directly to the liver. There, they're quickly converted into ketones—an efficient fuel source for both your body and brain. This makes MCT oil especially beneficial for those on ketogenic or low-carb diets, individuals with brain fog or energy dips, or anyone needing enhanced mental clarity and metabolic support. Even a small daily dose can help promote fat-burning, improve focus, and stabilize energy levels without the crash that comes from sugar or caffeine. Start with 1 teaspoon and gradually work up to 1–2 tablespoons per day to avoid digestive discomfort.

Reduced Insulin Levels: both keto and IF lower insulin levels, promoting insulin sensitivity and reducing the risk of insulin resistance, which is linked to type 2 diabetes and metabolic syndrome.

Increased Mental Clarity and Focus

Ketones as Brain Fuel: ketones provide a stable, efficient energy source for the brain, reducing brain fog and improving focus. This is why many people on keto report feeling more alert and mentally sharp. Our mitochondria prefer ketones as its main fuel source!

Neuroprotective Benefits: fasting triggers autophagy, a process of cellular repair and detoxification that removes damaged cells. This process can protect against neurodegenerative diseases and promote overall brain health.

Enhanced Energy and Reduced Cravings

Sustained Energy Levels: by relying on fat for fuel, energy levels become more consistent, avoiding the highs and lows associated with carb–heavy diets.

Reduced Cravings: ketosis can help reduce hunger and cravings. The addition of IF enhances this effect, as fasting helps stabilize hunger–regulating hormones like ghrelin.

Hormonal Balance and Longevity

Intermittent fasting (IF) plays a significant role in supporting hormonal balance, especially by boosting growth hormone levels. This hormone is vital for muscle maintenance, fat metabolism, cellular repair, and overall vitality. Additionally, both intermittent fasting and a ketogenic diet stimulate autophagy—the body's natural process of clearing out damaged cells and regenerating healthy ones. Autophagy is linked to reduced inflammation, slowed aging, and enhanced protection against chronic diseases, making it a powerful tool for longevity and anti–aging.

Improved Cardiovascular Health

One of the key benefits of combining keto and intermittent fasting is improved heart health. The ketogenic diet often raises HDL (the "good" cholesterol) and reduces triglyceride levels. When combined with intermittent fasting, it may also reduce small, dense LDL particles—the form most associated with plaque buildup and heart disease risk. It's important to understand that LDL itself is not harmful, it only becomes problematic when distorted by chronic oxidative stress and excessive sugar in the bloodstream. In such a state, LDL can no longer be properly processed by the liver, causing it to accumulate in arterial walls along with calcium and fibrin, contributing to plaque formation.

In addition, both keto and intermittent fasting may support blood pressure regulation by promoting better arterial flexibility and reducing systemic inflammation.

Tips for Combining Keto and Intermittent Fasting:
- **Ease into it**: begin with a ketogenic diet to allow your body to adapt to fat as its primary fuel source. Once your energy stabilizes, gradually extend the time between meals to implement intermittent fasting.
- **Stay hydrated**: both approaches can have diuretic effects, so it's essential to drink plenty of water and maintain proper electrolyte balance with minerals like sodium, potassium, and magnesium.
- **Prioritize nutrient density**: choose high-quality foods such as grassfed meats, organic vegetables, wild-caught fish, and healthy fats like avocados and coconut oil. These support optimal health, especially when eating fewer meals.
- **Listen to your body**: pay attention to energy levels, hunger cues, and digestion. Adjust your eating windows or macronutrient ratios as needed. If you find yourself getting hungry too soon, you may need to increase healthy fat intake, as fats help keep you fuller longer and stabilize blood sugar.

IMPORTANT NOTE:
Autophagy typically begins around 16 to 18 hours into a fast and acts like your body's internal cleanup crew—recycling old, dysfunctional cells and reducing toxic buildup. This process has been shown to support mental clarity, reduce anxiety, and boost overall cellular health. Exploring and understanding autophagy is highly recommended as it plays a major role in long-term wellness, metabolic balance, and emotional resilience.

By adopting a clean ketogenic lifestyle alongside intermittent fasting, you can experience profound improvements in energy, focus, metabolic flexibility, and overall health. However, as with any significant dietary shift, it's always wise to consult with a healthcare provider—especially if you're managing chronic conditions or taking medications.

Carnivore Diet

The carnivore diet focuses exclusively on animal-based foods such as meat, fish, eggs, and animal fats. It has gained popularity for its simplicity and potential therapeutic benefits, particularly for individuals with autoimmune or chronic inflammatory conditions. By eliminating plant-based foods, which often contain anti-nutrients like lectins, phytates, and oxalates, the carnivore diet may reduce gut irritation and promote improved nutrient absorption.

A major benefit of this way of eating is its nutrient density. Animal products are rich in highly bioavailable nutrients such as Vitamin B12, iron, zinc, omega-3 fatty acids, and fat-soluble vitamins like A, D, and K2. This nutrient concentration supports energy levels, hormonal balance, immune health, and overall vitality. In addition, the absence of carbohydrates and processed sugars helps stabilize blood sugar levels, reduce insulin spikes, and improve metabolic function, making this diet potentially beneficial for managing insulin resistance and type-2 diabetes.

Another compelling benefit is its anti–inflammatory potential. Many individuals with autoimmune conditions—such as rheumatoid arthritis, psoriasis, lupus, and Crohn's disease—have reported reduced symptoms and improved quality of life while on the carnivore diet. This is likely due to the removal of inflammatory foods, allergens, and irritants commonly found in grains, legumes, and processed foods. The diet also supports mental clarity, improved mood, and consistent energy, thanks to a stable supply of clean–burning fuel from fat and protein.

In terms of weight management, the carnivore diet naturally promotes satiety due to its high protein and fat content, helping reduce cravings and overeating without the need for calorie counting. Many find that by focusing on nutrient–dense foods like steak, eggs, and fish, they can effortlessly regulate their intake and maintain a leaner body composition.

For individuals with severe autoimmune or digestive issues, a more restricted version known as the Lion Diet is sometimes recommended. This approach includes only ruminant meats (such as beef and lamb), salt, and water. While highly restrictive, it serves as a powerful elimination diet that allows for a complete reset of the gut and immune system. Once symptoms improve, foods can be slowly reintroduced to identify personal triggers.

A Word on Sustainability of the Carnivore Diet

Personally, I don't believe a strict, all–meat carnivore diet is sustainable or ideal for long–term health over the course of many years. While it can be incredibly effective as a short–term therapeutic tool, especially for those dealing with autoimmune conditions, inflammation, or severe food sensitivities, the complete elimination of plant foods and dietary fiber may pose issues if continued indefinitely. There may be certain individuals who can sustain an all or mostly meat diet long term, but just word to the wise, just listen and be aware of your body and symptoms.

The human digestive system evolved to thrive on a diverse range of foods, including fibrous plant matter that supports the growth and maintenance of a healthy gut microbiome. Over time, individuals who eat exclusively animal products may lose key species of beneficial gut microbes—some of which rely on fermentable fibers (prebiotics) to survive. This microbial diversity is crucial for immune regulation, nutrient synthesis, and overall digestive health.

While our ancestors likely relied heavily on animal–based diets during times of scarcity or survival, especially in harsh climates—most anthropological evidence suggests that early humans consumed a variety of foods when available. In a survival scenario, red meat is arguably the most nutrient–dense and complete single food source, and many researchers agree it would be the ideal choice if stranded on an island.

That said, the goal should be metabolic flexibility, microbial balance, and long–term wellness, not just short–term symptom relief. Experts like Dr. William Davis and Mary Ruddick offer deeper insights into the importance of microbial health and how dietary variety, including targeted fiber and fermented foods, plays a role in maintaining a resilient gut ecosystem.

In short, a carnivore diet may be helpful during the healing phase, but reintroducing low–inflammatory, gut–supportive foods thoughtfully may be key for sustainable, lifelong health.

Mediterranean Diet

The Mediterranean diet is inspired by the traditional dietary patterns of cultures bordering the Mediterranean Sea. It emphasizes whole, minimally processed foods, including vegetables, fruits, whole grains, legumes, nuts, seeds, olive oil, and moderate amounts of fish, poultry, and dairy. Red meat is limited, and herbs and spices replace excessive salt, making meals both flavorful and health–conscious.

One of the primary benefits of the Mediterranean diet is its impact on heart health. Rich in monounsaturated fats (primarily from extra virgin olive oil) and omega-3 fatty acids (from fatty fish such as sardines and salmon), this eating pattern helps raise HDL (good) cholesterol, lower LDL oxidation, and reduce systemic inflammation—all of which contribute to a reduced risk of cardiovascular disease.

The diet also supports digestive health through a high intake of dietary fiber, promoting regular bowel movements, balanced blood sugar, and a healthy gut microbiome. In addition, its abundance of antioxidants—found in vegetables, berries, and nuts—helps combat oxidative stress and supports cellular repair throughout the body.

Cognitively, the Mediterranean diet (and lifestyle) is associated with a lower risk of neurodegenerative conditions such as Alzheimer's and dementia. This is due to the combination of anti-inflammatory foods, brain-nourishing omega-3s, and polyphenols that protect brain cells from age-related decline.

Unlike restrictive diets, the Mediterranean approach is flexible and enjoyable, making it more sustainable over the long term. It supports weight management by emphasizing satiating foods and discouraging overconsumption of processed snacks and sugars. The wide variety of flavors and textures keeps meals satisfying, helping to prevent diet fatigue.

Beyond physical health, this diet emphasizes lifestyle and community. Meals are often shared with loved ones, encouraging mindful eating, slower meals, and social connection—all of which are linked to improved emotional well-being and reduced stress. Often represented as a pyramid, the foundation of the Mediterranean diet includes daily physical activity and meaningful social interaction. From there, the diet is built on a base of plant foods and healthy fats, with seafood several times a week, modest portions of dairy and poultry, and occasional servings of red meat and sweets.

Both the carnivore and Mediterranean diets offer unique paths to health, depending on your individual needs and health challenges. The carnivore diet may benefit those with chronic inflammation, autoimmune conditions, or food sensitivities by simplifying the diet and reducing triggers. The Mediterranean diet, on the other hand, offers a balanced, anti–inflammatory lifestyle supported by decades of research. Whether you're looking to heal your gut, regulate blood sugar, manage weight, or simply feel better day to day, each of these dietary approaches has something valuable to offer when applied thoughtfully.

Ketovore Diet: A Balanced Hybrid of Keto and Carnivore

The *ketovore diet* is a strategic blend of the ketogenic and carnivore diets, focusing primarily on animal–based foods while maintaining a low carbohydrate intake. This approach emphasizes high–quality proteins and healthy fats—such as beef, lamb, poultry, eggs, fatty fish, and animal–derived fats—while allowing for small amounts of low–carb plant foods like leafy greens, herbs, or avocados. The goal is to stay in a state of ketosis, where the body uses fat and ketones as its primary fuel source instead of glucose.

One of the most significant benefits of the ketovore diet is its impact on metabolic health. By significantly lowering carbohydrate intake, it helps stabilize blood sugar levels, reduce insulin resistance, and support fat loss. This makes it especially valuable for individuals dealing with conditions like type–2 diabetes, obesity, or metabolic syndrome. Additionally, the high intake of healthy fats and protein leads to longer–lasting satiety, which naturally reduces hunger and cravings without needing to count calories.

The ketovore approach also promotes mental clarity and cognitive performance. Ketones are a clean–burning fuel for the brain, providing consistent energy without the crashes associated with blood sugar spikes. Many people report enhanced focus, reduced brain fog, and better emotional stability while following this diet. The emphasis on nutrient–dense, animal–based foods ensures abundant intake of essential vitamins and minerals like B vitamins, iron, zinc, omega–3s, and vitamin D—all of which support immune function, energy production, and hormonal balance.

Another advantage is its anti–inflammatory potential. By limiting or eliminating plant foods that may contain compounds like lectins, oxalates, and phytates (which can cause digestive distress or inflammation in sensitive individuals), the ketovore diet becomes an ideal tool for people dealing with autoimmune conditions, gut issues, or chronic inflammation. It also simplifies food choices, reducing decision fatigue and making healthy eating more sustainable over the long term.

Because it merges the structure of keto with the simplicity of carnivore, ketovore offers a flexible, sustainable approach to low–carb living. It allows for the benefits of ketosis while providing the freedom to include certain nutrient–rich plant foods as desired. The result is a satisfying, effective path toward better metabolism, improved cognitive health, and overall well–being.

Personal Reflection on Dietary Exploration

After over two decades of experimenting with a wide range of dietary approaches, including fasting, juice cleanses, ketogenic, carnivore, vegan, raw food, vegetarian, and ancestral hunter–gatherer diets, I've found that what works best for me is a hybrid of keto, carnivore, and Mediterranean principles. This approach emphasizes nutrient density, low–carb eating, and metabolic flexibility.

The key takeaway: there's no one–size–fits–all diet. It takes time, trial and error, and lifestyle refinement. But once you learn how your body responds, the rewards—mental sharpness, emotional stability, physical energy, and longevity—are well worth the commitment.

The Importance of Testosterone and the Modern Decline

Testosterone is a vital hormone, often referred to as the "master male hormone." It plays a critical role in muscle development, bone density, libido, mood regulation, fat distribution, and metabolic function. When testosterone is at optimal levels, men typically experience greater energy, stronger mental clarity, emotional stability, and resilience in the face of stress.

However, in recent decades, average testosterone levels in men have been declining at an alarming rate. Today's men, on average, have significantly lower testosterone than men of the same age just 50 years ago. This isn't merely a byproduct of aging; it's tied to modern lifestyle factors, most notably the rise in endocrine–disrupting chemicals found in our environment.

These substances—commonly found in plastics (like BPA), pesticides, household cleaners, personal care products, and even some food additives—interfere with the body's hormone signaling. When combined with poor diet, lack of exercise, chronic stress, and inadequate sleep, these environmental factors can contribute to low testosterone and related symptoms such as fatigue, depression, low libido, increased body fat, and muscle loss.

Reversing this trend starts with eliminating or reducing exposure to hormone disruptors, prioritizing nutrient–rich diets like keto, ketovore, or Mediterranean, and supporting lifestyle habits that naturally optimize testosterone—such as resistance training, deep sleep, sun exposure (vitamin D), and stress reduction.

Healing from the Inside Out: The Power of the GAPS Diet

This subject truly deserves its own dedicated chapter—because it's that important. The Gut and Psychology Syndrome (GAPS) Diet has changed countless lives and continues to offer hope to those dealing with chronic illness, mental health challenges, and stubborn digestive disorders. It's a powerful nutritional protocol designed to heal and seal the gut lining, restore microbiome balance, and reduce systemic inflammation—an approach that's helped many when conventional medicine fell short.

Before we go any further, I want to immediately spotlight one of the pioneers of this protocol in the West: Dr. Natasha Campbell–McBride. She's a neurologist and nutritionist who developed the GAPS Diet out of necessity for her own child, and her work has since guided thousands of practitioners, parents, and individuals around the world. If you're chronically ill, caring for someone who is, or are a therapist or health coach looking to understand the gut–brain–immune connection more deeply, **I strongly urge you to read her books**, especially *Gut and Psychology Syndrome* and *Gut and Physiology Syndrome*.

Now, let's dive into the fundamentals of the GAPS Diet, and why it is so critical, especially in modern times, when skyrocketing rates of autoimmune disease, food intolerances, ADHD, autism spectrum disorders, IBS, depression, and anxiety often share a common root: **a compromised gut**.

The GAPS diet was developed by Dr. Natasha Campbell–McBride as a therapeutic nutritional protocol designed to heal the gut lining and restore the balance of gut flora. It consists of 3 main Phases: intro to GAPS, GAPS full diet and phasing out of GAPS into a healthy everyday "GAPS–style" diet. Most people who go down this route will be on some form of this GAPS style diet for years.

The GAPS diet is primarily used for individuals dealing with a range of neurological and digestive conditions such as autism, ADHD, depression, anxiety, autoimmune issues, and chronic inflammation. The underlying principle is that many of these disorders stem from a damaged digestive system, particularly a "leaky gut," where toxins, undigested food particles, and pathogens pass into the bloodstream and negatively affect brain function and immune regulation.

The diet emphasizes removing hard–to–digest and inflammatory foods while introducing nutrient–rich, easily digestible meals that promote gut healing. It starts with an Introductory Phase, which includes bone broths, boiled meats, fermented vegetables, and simple cooked vegetables. Gradually, more foods are added, such as eggs, ghee, stews, and eventually raw vegetables and fruits. The Full GAPS Diet includes a wider variety of whole, unprocessed foods but still avoids grains, processed sugar, and most dairy except for fermented forms.

This approach is not just about managing symptoms; it is aimed at rebuilding the gut from the inside out. A healed gut means fewer toxins reaching the brain, better nutrient absorption, and more balanced neurotransmitter production. This is especially important for individuals with anxiety, PTSD, or neurological challenges, as the gut–brain connection plays a central role in mood regulation, stress resilience, and cognitive clarity.

Beyond mental health, the GAPS diet supports the immune system by improving the integrity of the intestinal lining and reducing chronic inflammation, which is often at the root of autoimmune issues and fatigue. Though the diet can be demanding and requires patience, many who follow it experience significant improvements in digestion, mental clarity, emotional balance, and overall vitality. In essence, the GAPS diet is about nourishing the body deeply and creating the internal environment necessary for long–term healing and emotional stability.

The GAPS Intro Diet is the first phase of the Gut and Psychology Syndrome program and is designed to gently start healing the gut lining and calming inflammation. There are 6 stages of the INTRO phase.

It begins with very simple, easy–to–digest foods like homemade meat or fish bone broths, soft–cooked vegetables, boiled meats, and fermented foods like sauerkraut juice. These foods help soothe the digestive tract, support the growth of good bacteria, and begin sealing up a "leaky gut." The Intro Diet is done in 6 stages, slowly adding more foods like egg yolks, ghee, cooked vegetables, and eventually meats, stews, and fermented dairy like homemade yogurt or kefir. Each stage is meant to be personalized based on how your body responds, moving slowly if there are reactions and progressing when digestion improves. Though strict at first, the Intro Diet is one of the most powerful parts of the GAPS program for reducing symptoms like bloating, flatulence, IBS, digestive disturbances, food sensitivities, brain fog, physical pain, auto–immunity and immune system disfunction, emotional instability and almost every other issue that comes from the dysfunctional "leaky gut."

That's about as far as we'll go here with the GAPS Diet for now, but I want to leave you with a personal note:

At the time of this writing, I'm in the final stages of the GAPS Intro Diet, nearly completing all six stages in just under two months. Dr. Natasha Campbell–McBride emphasizes that everyone progresses at their own pace. Some move quickly, others more slowly, depending on their level of gut damage and overall health. Because I had already been following a very strict keto and carnivore diet for the past two years, I didn't have to overhaul everything—just make strategic changes, add some things, remove others, and commit fully to the process.

After about six weeks, I've been nearly zero–carb and zero–sugar, and I can confidently say: I feel amazing. My brain is sharper. My energy is steady throughout the day. And most importantly, my body is finally starting to function the way it's supposed to.

I've battled chronic infections for years, which made me feel like I was constantly dragging myself through life—exhausted, inflamed, and foggy. Since starting GAPS, I've noticed a major shift. I'm no longer reacting to foods like I used to, and that's had a direct impact on lowering my cortisol and calming my nervous system. I'm sleeping better, thinking more clearly, and no longer walking around feeling like I got hit by a truck.

So yes, I highly recommend looking into this diet if any of what I'm describing feels familiar to you. We're living in a world filled with toxins, chemicals, processed foods, and stressors that are silently destroying our guts, immune systems, and mental health. Leaky gut and gut dysbiosis are not fringe topics anymore—they're real, and they're often at the root of so many health issues.

If a lightbulb went off for you while reading this section, follow that spark. Pick up one of Dr. Campbell-McBride's books, watch some of the countless GAPS success stories on YouTube, and consider starting this journey for yourself. It takes effort, yes. But a little discipline and sacrifice now can transform your life for the better. Work hard for a while—and it will absolutely pay off.

Now, let's shift gears and get into something just as critical: A foundational understanding of neurotransmitters. Your nutrition and lifestyle directly shape your brain chemistry—and stress? That's not just emotional. It's biochemical. Let's break it down.

GABA (Gamma-Aminobutyric Acid)

GABA is your brain's main calming neurotransmitter, acting like a natural brake on stress and overthinking. It helps slow down neural activity, promoting relaxation, sleep, and anxiety relief. People with PTSD often have low GABA levels, making it harder to settle the mind and body. **Nutrition tip:** magnesium, Vitamin B6, and fermented foods can help support GABA production. Create a calming evening routine with deep breathing, magnesium-rich foods, and screen-free time to promote GABA and ease anxiety.

Glutamate

Glutamate is the main excitatory neurotransmitter in the brain, involved in learning and memory. While necessary for brain function, too much glutamate (or poor clearance) can lead to neurotoxicity, hypervigilance, and anxiety—common in PTSD. Balancing it with GABA is key. **Nutrition tip:** limit processed foods and other food toxins (pesticides, additives, etc.) and increase antioxidants (like Vitamin C, zinc, and omega–3s) to prevent glutamate overload.

Serotonin

Serotonin regulates mood, sleep, digestion, and a sense of safety and well–being. It's often depleted in PTSD, contributing to depression, insomnia, and emotional instability. About 90% of serotonin is made in the gut, so healthy digestion is critical. **Nutrition tip:** tryptophan–rich foods (turkey, eggs, salmon), B vitamins, and probiotics can support gut–brain health. GAPS diet and leaky gut problems are especially connected to serotonin because of the gut–brain connection. The gut cannot make it properly and adequately if it's dysfunctional. Get outside in the morning sun, eat tryptophan–rich foods like eggs or turkey, and nourish your gut with GAPS style meals and probiotics to naturally boost serotonin.

Dopamine

Dopamine is tied to motivation, pleasure, reward, and focus. In PTSD, dopamine pathways can become disrupted, leading to emotional numbness, low motivation, and trouble concentrating. Supporting dopamine helps rebuild drive and joy. **Nutrition tip:** tyrosine–rich foods (beef, eggs, dairy, organic only almonds), and Vitamin B6, help fuel dopamine production. Set meaningful goals and fulfill them, enjoy protein–rich GAPS style meals, and practice gratitude or exercise daily to your level, to stimulate dopamine and restore motivation.

Norepinephrine (Noradrenaline)

This is your alertness and stress response chemical. It increases heart rate, focus, and energy during a threat. In PTSD, it's often chronically elevated in a false alarm status (as you read earlier on), causing hypervigilance, poor sleep, and heightened startle response. **Nutrition tip:** stabilizing blood sugar with balanced meals, supporting adrenal health with vitamin C, B5, and reducing stimulants like caffeine, alcohol and any processed foods help a more balanced hormone release. Practice deep belly breathing, vagus nerve exercises, or gentle yoga and stretching to shift from fight–or–flight into rest–and–digest mode. Poor or inconsistent sleep increases both norepinephrine and epinephrine. Set a calming bedtime routine and aim for 7 to 9 hours per night.

Epinephrine (Adrenaline)

Closely related to norepinephrine, epinephrine drives the "fight or flight" response. It spikes during trauma or perceived danger. In PTSD, your body may overreact to non–dangerous cues. Managing adrenaline is about calming the system through breathing, movement, and nutrition that supports adrenal recovery (e.g., adaptogens, healthy fats, and minerals like magnesium and potassium). Practice deep belly breathing, vagus nerve exercises, or gentle yoga and stretching to shift from fight–or–flight into rest–and–digest mode. Use grounding activities like walking barefoot and blood sugar–stabilizing meals to help lower chronic adrenaline surges.

Everything we talk about in this book relates to this as well, especially cognitive behavior therapy. Herbs like ashwagandha, rhodiola, and holy basil help buffer the body's stress response and support adrenal balance. I've used these herbs in the past but do your own research to make sure they're right for you. Meaningful connection and emotional safety can also help calm the body's stress axis and support a more balanced hormone release.

Cortisol

Cortisol is your main stress hormone, regulating energy, blood sugar, and inflammation. In PTSD, cortisol may be too high (constant stress) or too low (burnout). It disrupts sleep, digestion, and mood. **Nutrition tip**: avoid sugar spikes, eat protein first with every meal, then other foods after, and support with omega–3s and B vitamins. Support your circadian rhythm with regular sleep, stress–reducing practices like meditation, and nutrient-dense meals that include healthy fats and B vitamins.

Cortisol and blood sugar are also closely linked and can have a significant impact on anxiety and stress. When blood sugar drops too low, it signals the body to release cortisol to raise glucose levels. Cortisol works to convert stored energy into glucose, ensuring that the brain and body have enough fuel. However, this increase in cortisol can lead to feelings of anxiety, restlessness, and irritability, as the body enters a "fight-or-flight" mode in response to perceived stress.

Chronically high cortisol levels, which can result from prolonged stress or irregular blood sugar control, contribute to a vicious cycle of anxiety. High cortisol levels also impact blood sugar regulation by reducing the effectiveness of insulin, causing glucose levels to fluctuate. This can create a pattern of energy crashes and spikes, which often intensifies feelings of stress and anxiety. Additionally, high cortisol can lead to symptoms like insomnia, increased heart rate, and irritability—all of which exacerbate anxiety.

Managing blood sugar with regular, balanced meals can help stabilize glucose levels, which, in turn, reduces unnecessary spikes in cortisol. Practices from this book in later chapters, like mindfulness, deep breathing, and regular physical activity also play a vital role in keeping cortisol levels in check. Together, these strategies can support both blood sugar stability and emotional resilience, breaking the cycle of high cortisol and its effect on stress and anxiety.

Endorphins

Endorphins are the body's natural painkillers and mood boosters—released during exercise, laughter, and positive social interaction. PTSD often leads to low endorphin activity, which contributes to emotional numbness or chronic pain. Boost naturally with movement, sunlight, physical touch, and foods like dark chocolate. Some say spicy foods but if you're healing leaky gut, steer away from spicy foods for a little while. Move your body with joyful exercise, laugh often, spend time in nature and connect with loved ones.

Oxytocin

Known as the bonding and safety hormone, oxytocin helps you feel connected, loved, and secure. PTSD can blunt oxytocin responses, making it hard to trust or feel safe with others. Nutrition isn't a direct driver here, but physical touch, healthy relationships, meditation, and some probiotics (like *lactobacillus reuteri*) can help elevate it naturally. Foster safe, meaningful connection with loved ones and friends through hugs, time with pets, or shared meals to raise oxytocin and rebuild trust and emotional safety.

Probiotics

Probiotics are probably the most IMPORTANT part of our health, especially in our modern–day toxic world. Probiotics are beneficial bacteria and yeasts that help maintain a healthy gut microbiome, which is directly connected to your brain and nervous system through what is called the gut–brain axis. This connection is crucial when you're working with PTSD, anxiety, chronic stress, autoimmunity, and chronic illness. Many people don't realize that the gut influences not only digestion, but also inflammation, neurotransmitter production, immune response, and mood regulation.

When your gut lining becomes compromised, a state known as leaky gut, undigested particles and toxins can leak into the bloodstream, triggering systemic inflammation and worsening autoimmune and anxiety–related symptoms. For example, because of the similarity between the shape of gluten peptides and proteins found in certain bacteria, when a gluten peptide leaks into the bloodstream through the gut, this can trigger the immune system because the body can't tell the difference between attacking the bacteria versus the gluten peptide. Restoring gut health through probiotics is a critical step in calming this cascade and helping the nervous system find a more regulated state.

Lactobacillus strains are among the most well-studied probiotics. They play an important role in breaking down food and producing lactic acid, which maintains an acidic gut environment that discourages harmful bacteria. They also help regulate immune responses and support the production of GABA, a calming neurotransmitter that is often depleted in those with PTSD and chronic anxiety. People with stress-related gut issues, such as IBS or bloating, often benefit from increasing *Lactobacillus* species in their system.

Bifidobacteria are one of the first bacterial groups to colonize the human gut and are vital for maintaining gut barrier integrity, critical in preventing or healing leaky gut. They also help digest complex carbohydrates, produce short-chain fatty acids (which fuel the gut lining), and modulate immune responses. In cases of autoimmunity and chronic illness, having healthy levels of *Bifidobacteria* can make a huge difference in calming systemic inflammation. These strains are also linked to improved mood and emotional resilience through their influence on serotonin and other neurotransmitters.

Lactobacillus reuteri has emerged as a particularly interesting strain for those working on emotional healing and nervous system regulation. It not only supports gut barrier integrity and reduces gut inflammation, but also promotes the release of oxytocin, the "bonding hormone." Studies suggest that *L. reuteri* supplementation can help improve social connection, reduce anxiety, and even promote self-compassion, which is often a core wound in PTSD and trauma survivors. For those dealing with emotional isolation or social withdrawal, this strain is worth exploring.

Saccharomyces boulardii is a beneficial yeast, but it plays a key role in gut health, especially for those recovering from gut infections, antibiotic use, or chronic inflammation. *S. boulardii* helps restore microbial balance, supports immune regulation, and helps reduce gut permeability (leaky gut). This is especially valuable for people with autoimmune conditions, as a leaky gut often triggers flares and worsens symptoms. It also helps calm inflammatory responses that can feed into anxiety and nervous system dysregulation.

Supporting your gut microbiome is not just about better digestion, it is directly tied to mental health, immune balance, inflammation, and overall resilience. For anyone dealing with PTSD, anxiety, chronic illness, or autoimmune issues, incorporating targeted probiotics is one of the most foundational and powerful tools for healing both body and mind. For more information, I recommend looking at the work done by Dr. William Davis, Dr. Natasha Campbell McBride, and Mary Ruddick.

The way I'm getting probiotics right now is through homemade yogurt made with *L. reuteri*, *Bifidobacteria*, and other *Lactobacillus* strains (plus many more strains found naturally in organic/grassfed kefir). Sometimes I'll just have a small amount of straight kefir once a day. Let me tell you, homemade yogurt is leagues above store–bought yogurt—they're not even in the same category. With homemade yogurt, you get far more beneficial bacteria (comparable to taking a small handful of probiotic capsules) without any added sugar or other harmful additives.

Another way I get probiotics is through raw fermented vegetables, especially sauerkraut. I even put a little sauerkraut juice into my meat broth (not to be confused with bone broth). First thing in the morning, I drink meat broth, which comes from cooking whole meat with bones, joints, and skin. After cooling it down to warm (not hot), I add a small spoon of MCT oil and some sauerkraut juice. You don't want it to be too hot, as that would damage the MCT oil and probiotics. I also eat fermented veggies and sauerkraut with meals throughout the day. Having this first thing in the morning is incredibly healing for the gut lining, it gives your body and gut exactly what they need to start the day and support healing. If the broth tastes too bland, I'll simply add a pinch of sea salt to bring it to life.

One more reason I eat yogurt, fermented veggies, and drink fermented juices is because our bodies need those beneficial bacteria not just in the gut, but throughout the entire digestive system, starting from the oral cavity and throat all the way down. Different bacteria support different areas, but overall, it's very important to regularly bring these good bacteria into the system through food and drink. Drinking them down helps repopulate and support the natural balance of your entire digestive tract, not just the lower gut—giving your whole system what it needs to stay strong and resilient.

Homemade yogurt, especially when fermented using specific probiotic strains like *L. reuteri, Lactobacillus gasseri, Bifidobacterium infantis*, offers a wide range of health benefits, as extensively discussed by Dr. William Davis and other leading voices in functional medicine. This powerful food helps restore and optimize the gut microbiome, which is often damaged by antibiotics, stress, processed foods, and environmental toxins like glyphosate. By reintroducing beneficial bacteria, homemade yogurt plays a critical role in repairing the gut barrier, reducing inflammation, and supporting overall digestive health. Certain strains, such as *L. reuteri*, are known to increase oxytocin levels, a hormone associated with emotional bonding, deep sleep, and stress relief. This can lead to better REM sleep, calmer moods, and enhanced emotional resilience.

Additionally, homemade yogurt has been shown to support skin health by improving hydration and collagen production, which may reduce wrinkles and improve elasticity. It also benefits metabolic function by improving insulin sensitivity, lowering blood glucose, and even supporting weight loss—particularly when using strains like *L. gasseri*, which have been linked to reduced abdominal fat. For individuals struggling with immune dysregulation or autoimmune conditions, homemade yogurt can help strengthen immune responses and reduce flare-ups by restoring microbial diversity and mucosal immunity in the gut.

Moreover, the gut–brain axis plays a significant role in mental health, and regular consumption of targeted yogurt strains can help enhance the production of neurotransmitters like serotonin, dopamine, and GABA, leading to clearer thinking, less anxiety, and improved emotional regulation. Some strains, like *S. boulardii*, also support the resolution of yeast overgrowth, diarrhea, and digestive infections, making homemade yogurt a versatile tool for gut repair. For those recovering from conditions like small intestinal bacterial overgrowth (SIBO) or chronic dysbiosis, this kind of therapeutic yogurt may become a cornerstone of healing.

The beauty of homemade yogurt lies in its customizability; you can tailor the bacterial strains to your specific health goals. Whether you're looking to support mood, digestion, skin, metabolic function, or immunity, there's likely a combination that fits your needs. And with its rich nutrient profile and live cultures, this isn't just food, it's medicine.

Plastics and Xenoestrogens:

A major contributor to declining testosterone levels is exposure to xenoestrogens, which are synthetic chemicals that mimic estrogen in the body. These compounds are commonly found in plastics, personal care products, pesticides, and even in the lining of canned foods. When plastics are exposed to heat, they can leach chemicals like Bisphenol A (BPA) and phthalates into food and beverages. Once ingested, these chemicals mimic estrogen, binding to hormone receptors and disrupting the body's endocrine system. This interference can reduce the body's natural testosterone production, leading to hormonal imbalances that can have significant health consequences over time. The effects are compounded by the fact that xenoestrogens don't simply degrade or disappear; they accumulate in the body over years of exposure, adding to the overall burden on hormonal health.

Beyond plastics, other aspects of the modern lifestyle contribute to lower testosterone levels. Chronic stress is a big factor. When the body is under prolonged stress, it releases high levels of cortisol, a hormone that, when consistently elevated, can inhibit testosterone production. Additionally, poor sleep quality or insufficient sleep can lower testosterone production, as most testosterone is produced during deep sleep.

Diet also plays a role in testosterone levels. A diet high in processed foods, sugar, and trans fats can lead to weight gain, particularly around the abdomen, which is associated with lower testosterone. Excess body fat increases the enzyme aromatase, which converts testosterone into estrogen, further contributing to hormonal imbalances. Sedentary behavior also has a negative impact; men who don't engage in regular physical activity, particularly strength training, tend to have lower testosterone levels. Exercise stimulates testosterone production, so without it, testosterone levels are likely to decrease.

In addition to plastics, there is increasing exposure to other environmental toxins and pesticides that contain endocrine disruptors. Many common pesticides used in conventional farming contain chemicals that disrupt hormone function, impacting testosterone levels. Foods grown with these pesticides can carry residues that, over time, contribute to a man's exposure to estrogenic compounds.

The decline in testosterone levels is not an inevitable part of aging but a reflection of our modern environment and lifestyle choices. By becoming aware of these factors, you can take proactive steps to protect your hormonal health. This can include choosing products free from harmful chemicals, eating a diet rich in whole foods, managing stress effectively, prioritizing sleep, and engaging in regular physical activity.

Exposure in women has been linked to a range of health issues, particularly concerning fertility and hormonal balance. Again, the xenoestrogens found in plastics, personal care products, and pesticides, disrupt the body's endocrine system by binding to estrogen receptors, leading to an excess of estrogen relative to other hormones. This imbalance can contribute to reproductive issues like irregular menstrual cycles, heavy periods, and conditions such as polycystic ovary syndrome (PCOS) and endometriosis, all of which can negatively impact fertility. Additionally, xenoestrogens are associated with earlier onset of puberty, as they can prompt premature hormonal changes in young girls, which is a concerning trend seen over recent decades.

Women exposed to xenoestrogens may also experience symptoms of estrogen dominance, such as bloating, mood swings, and breast tenderness. Over time, these chemicals can increase the risk of hormone–related cancers, including breast and ovarian cancers. By taking steps to minimize exposure, such as avoiding plastic containers, choosing natural personal care products, and opting for organic foods, women can better support their hormonal health. These changes help reduce the burden of xenoestrogens on the body, promoting a healthier hormonal balance and protecting reproductive health for the long term.

Taking steps to reduce exposure to xenoestrogens can significantly support hormonal health and fertility. This includes choosing natural, hormone–free personal care products and makeup, as these are direct sources of exposure. Selecting products without parabens, phthalates, and other synthetic chemicals helps protect the skin and body from these hormone disruptors. Opting for glass or stainless steel over plastic containers, using organic produce, and filtering drinking water can also help reduce exposure.

By making these lifestyle changes, you can minimize your interaction with xenoestrogens, supporting healthier hormonal balance and reproductive health. Growing awareness of these risks emphasizes the importance of choosing safer, natural alternatives to protect health, both now and for future generations.

Takeaways from Chapter 3

- **GAPS Diet**: please look more into this and get the support that most people need from this lifestyle. I can't stress enough about how much this diet has helped me.
- Nutrition is extremely important in this day and age. Food is medicine!
- Malnourishment is a real thing even here in the United States because of the ultra–processed foods and peoples' metabolic and digestive disorders
- You **NEED** to supplement (with the supervision of a medical professional as appropriate) with high–quality and third–party tested supplement. Unless you are eating meat "from nose to tail" which most are not, you probably need supplementation. If you are on a carnivore diet or are limited to beef only, you most likely need supplementation.
- Important supplements to remember: Omega 3s, B vitamins, magnesium, Vitamin D3/K2, zinc, electrolytes, and sea salt from healthy and quality sources.
- Getting on the right low carb diet that works for you is important and (at least) a great start.
- Eating organic food, especially in the United States is important because of glyphosate and other pesticides and herbicides.
- Nitric Oxide supplementation can be important for high blood pressure and chronic conditions, especially lung issues and infections. Dr. Nathan Bryan states that people on ventilators with infections were all much too low on nitric oxide.
- Testosterone is important for everyone, especially for men, in this modern day.
- Plastics = bad. Plastics are all around us, in the kitchen, every part of the house, in the food, water, air, polyester and other synthetic clothing. Consider switching out plastic when possible.
- Bromine, fluoride and chlorine are all around us as well, use your secret weapon, iodine!
- High cortisol from chronic stress and poor sleep, combined with frequent blood sugar spikes and crashes, can throw your

hormones, stress levels, and anxiety into chaos—leaving you bouncing around like kids in a bouncy house with no off switch.
- **If you don't take much of anything from the nutrition chapter, then please remember 2 things: 1) fix the leaky gut and gut microbiome with GAPS and/or Dr. William Davis protocols, and 2) look into a low carb, keto/ carnivore lifestyle. Gut Microbes and Nutritional deficiencies are causing people so much mental and physical distress.**

Chapter 4
Doctor, Doctor Give Me the News

"The art of medicine consists of amusing the patient while nature cures the disease."
— *Voltaire*

This might seem like a detour but trust me, the information in this chapter could be more important than you realize. It certainly was for me. For years, I lived with a range of strange and exhausting physical sensations that left me feeling confused, anxious, and at times, completely defeated. I didn't know what was going on in my body. The symptoms were real, but the answers, they felt just out of reach. Finally taking the time to explore what was—and just as importantly, what *wasn't*—happening in my body brought me some much-needed clarity. Even ruling out certain conditions gave me peace of mind and a bit of ground to stand on.

Looking back, I realize how little I understood my own symptoms during those years. It was like trying to navigate a storm blindfolded. But getting a few simple, routine tests through my doctor changed everything. The results didn't magically fix all my issues, but they gave me something powerful: *clarity*. And with clarity came calm. Knowing that some of my systems were functioning normally helped lower my stress and allowed me to focus on healing rather than guessing.

At one point, I even got tested for Lyme disease. Several people in my life who tested positive said, "you know, what you're going through really sounds like Lyme." That planted a seed of fear and added another layer of anxiety to an already full plate. I finally got tested, and thankfully, I was negative. That one answer lifted a heavy weight off my shoulders. Years of doubt, speculation, and uncertainty were replaced with a sense of relief. If you're carrying a similar burden, wondering what might be going on in your body, I encourage you—*don't wait*. Get checked. Even if it's just to cross something off the list, the clarity alone is worth it.

I also want to say this clearly: **I'm not against pharmaceuticals.** I believe in starting with natural healing methods whenever possible, nutrition, lifestyle changes, supplements, and detox, but if those don't bring relief within a reasonable timeframe, get the support you need. There is no shame in using medications when appropriate. Often, the best approach is a blend of both: using conventional medicine as a bridge while working on deeper, long-term healing through natural means.

As for autoimmune disorders, they're a massive topic, too big to fully explore here, but we did cover a solid amount in the previous chapter. I want you to know this: you're not alone. Many practitioners now specialize in autoimmune issues, and there's a growing number of people sharing their journeys openly. YouTube and similar platforms are full of incredibly valuable insights, stories, and education from real people who have walked this road and found answers, sometimes after years of searching.

Don't lose hope. Answers do exist. And every step you take to understand what's happening inside your body is a step toward reclaiming your health. One of the first steps is to learn about what's going on in your body.

Cholesterol: The Truth Behind the Myth

This topic deserves its own spotlight, not just because it's so misunderstood, but because it's one of the areas I've personally researched the most—and what I've uncovered may surprise you.

Let's start with a bit of history.

The narrative that cholesterol and dietary fat are the villains behind heart disease largely originated in the 1950s with Ancel Keys, an American physiologist. Keys became widely known for his *Seven Countries Study*, which claimed to show a direct link between saturated fat intake and coronary heart disease. His research profoundly influenced public health policy and shaped dietary guidelines for decades. However, the foundation of that research has since been widely criticized—and rightfully so.

Here's the issue: Keys selectively used data from countries that supported his theory and ignored others that didn't. Nations like France and Switzerland, where people consumed high levels of saturated fat but had low rates of heart disease, were conveniently left out. This cherry-picking of evidence created a misleading narrative— one that demonized dietary fat and cholesterol, while pushing the now infamous low-fat, high-carb diet.

As a result, natural fats like butter, eggs, and red meat were wrongly vilified, and processed, sugary foods flooded the market under the guise of being "heart-healthy." It wasn't until decades later that independent researchers began to dig deeper and found that the science behind this fat-phobia was not only flawed, but manipulated.

One of the most shocking revelations was that the sugar industry funded studies in the 1960s and '70s that intentionally shifted the blame away from sugar and onto dietary fat. Recently uncovered internal documents revealed that sugar lobbyists paid researchers to downplay the role of sugar in heart disease. But the damage was already done. Fat was demonized, sugar was exonerated, and the consequences were widespread.

Today, we know better. Modern research shows that dietary cholesterol has a minimal impact on blood cholesterol levels in most people. It's not cholesterol or saturated fat that's driving the heart disease epidemic—it's chronic inflammation, insulin resistance, and a diet loaded with processed carbs and refined sugars.

The cholesterol myth is finally starting to unravel. Real, whole foods like eggs, grass–fed meat, and animal fats are making a comeback. People are waking up to the fact that food *quality* matters far more than targeting or avoiding a single nutrient.

Let's clear up some key points.

The narrative around "high cholesterol" and "bad LDL" has been oversimplified and, in many cases, misinformed. Low–Density Lipoprotein (LDL) is your delivery truck for cholesterol and fat–soluble nutrients throughout the body. LDL is not "bad." The issue arises when LDL becomes small, dense, and oxidized—typically due to lifestyle factors like processed food consumption, smoking, poor sleep, and high stress. These damaged particles can linger in the bloodstream and cause micro–tears (lesions) in artery walls, which then attract calcium, fibrin, and other materials that build up as plaque—a combination of hardened cholesterol, damaged lipoproteins, and calcium.

When arterial lesions form, LDL and cholesterol rush in to help heal them—like ambulances going to a crash site. But if you're continuously consuming processed foods, sugar, alcohol, not getting enough sunlight, insufficient sleep, and not exercising, those lesions don't heal, and more cholesterol keeps building up. Additionally, triglycerides, a type of lipid often elevated by poor diet, are major contributors to this entire process. Triglycerides contribute to inflammation, which depletes magnesium (and other nutrients) and causes further buildup. This eventually creates plaque (atherosclerosis), which can cause blood clots, heart attacks, strokes and other medical emergencies.

High–Density Lipoprotein (HDL) is your cleanup crew. HDL helps remove excess cholesterol from the bloodstream and transport it back to the liver for recycling. A healthy balance between LDL and HDL is what really matters. So, don't just look at total cholesterol. A far more telling marker is your triglyceride–to–HDL ratio. Simply divide your triglyceride number by your HDL. A ratio below 2 is good, while 1.8 or lower is ideal. A ratio above 3 is considered too high and suggests poor metabolic health. If all you're looking at is the total cholesterol without evaluating your numbers further, significant health issues can be missed.

Let's break down inflammation and oxidative stress.

The real enemy is not cholesterol; it's oxidative stress and inflammation. These are the real root causes behind the epidemic of cardiovascular disease, heart attacks, diabetes, and other metabolic disorders, not cholesterol. Oxidative stress and inflammation are driven by ultra–processed foods, environmental toxins, sugar overload, poor sleep, and chronic stress— it's a perfect storm of modern lifestyle factors that wreak havoc on the body.

Our systems are under constant assault from excessive sugar and high–carbohydrate diets, toxins from the environment, air, water, food, household products and unnatural objects that release VOC's and plastics. This leads to chronically elevated insulin levels and metabolic dysfunction. Add to that dysregulated immune and nervous systems, depleted and harmful gut microbes, chronic inflammation, and we have a recipe for widespread disease.

Again, one of the most dangerous consequences of this internal chaos is the distortion of small, dense LDL particles. These damaged particles are not the problem in and of themselves—they're a *symptom* of oxidative stress and cellular breakdown. When they become oxidized due to poor diet, environmental toxins, trans fats, and industrial seed oils (like canola, corn, and soybean oil), the body can no longer properly process them. Instead of being recycled by the liver, they circulate and get trapped in the arterial walls, causing micro–tears, inflammation, and eventually dangerous plaque buildup. Bottom line: When LDL becomes oxidized, it's no longer the delivery truck, it's a problem.

Alcohol and smoking are also massive contributors to this oxidative burden, particularly in the liver and blood vessels. These substances weaken the body's ability to manage stress, repair damage, and detoxify properly, which amplifies the effects of poor nutrition and metabolic overload.

Let's talk about what you can do.

Whenever possible, avoid processed foods. Processed foods not only disrupt cholesterol balance but also rob your body of vital nutrients and harm your gut microbiome. Make other lifestyle changes as well to tamp down that internal storm. Incorporating key nutrients like Vitamin D3, Vitamin K2, and magnesium helps prevent this calcification by guiding calcium into the bones where it belongs and keeping it out of arteries.

You don't have to avoid using fat, but what you use matters. Animal fats are incredibly stable and safe for cooking. Fats from pasture–raised animals (like tallow, lard, butter, and ghee) remain structurally stable under heat. In contrast, industrial seed oils—canola, corn, soybean, cottonseed, vegetable oil—are already oxidized before you even use them. When heated, they produce harmful compounds that are highly inflammatory and damaging at the cellular level. Even olive oil should be used with caution as heating it to high temperatures renders any health benefits moot. Even though trans fats have been "banned" in some countries, they still sneak into our food supply under different names. Many packaged and fast foods still contain small amounts that, over time, accumulate and contribute to systemic inflammation.

It's time to reclaim cholesterol's reputation and understand its true role in the body. Cholesterol is essential for hormone production, brain health, cell membrane integrity, and Vitamin D synthesis. Without it, we cannot thrive. Let's remember the bigger lesson here: science must remain transparent and free from corporate influence. We must stay curious, ask questions, and challenge long–held assumptions, especially when it comes to our health.

Here's the big picture: your body isn't broken, it's responding to the environment it's being given. When you give it the right tools, it can begin to heal.

Let's be clear: **cholesterol is not the villain.** In fact, cholesterol is part of the body's natural repair system—it rushes in to help heal damage caused by inflammation and oxidative stress. When cholesterol is found at the scene of the problem, it's not the criminal; it's the medic.

It's time to shift the narrative and focus on the *true culprits* behind today's health crisis: sugar, refined carbs, processed foods, toxic fats, chronic stress, environmental toxins, alcohol, and smoking—not cholesterol. Cholesterol has been trying to save our lives, not end them.

Here's the caveat...

If you've recently transitioned to a keto or carnivore diet and notice that your cholesterol numbers have increased, don't panic. This is actually a common occurrence—and one that doesn't necessarily indicate a problem. What's more important than your *total* cholesterol number is your metabolic health as a whole. If your fasting insulin, triglyceride–to–HDL ratio, and Vitamin D levels are all in good ranges, you're likely on solid ground.

Personally, I feel confident in my health based on these markers, and I encourage you to take a similar holistic approach. Of course, I'm *not* a doctor, just someone passionate about nutrition who's done a lot of research and learning over the years. Much of what I've learned comes directly from doctors, cardiologists and experts I follow closely, and the good news is: this isn't hidden or secret knowledge. It's *foundational metabolic science* that we've known for decades, but don't hear enough about.

Dr. William Davis, cardiologist and author of *Wheat Belly* and *Super Gut*, emphasizes that total cholesterol alone is a poor indicator of heart disease risk. He explains that focusing on total cholesterol misses the bigger picture of metabolic health and can lead to unnecessary fear or medication. According to Dr. Davis, what truly matters is the type and size of cholesterol particles, particularly small, dense LDL particles, which are far more atherogenic (plaque–forming) than large, fluffy LDL. He encourages patients and readers to look at advanced lipid testing, such as lipoprotein particle counts (e.g., ApoB or LDL–P) and the triglyceride–to–HDL ratio, which are much better predictors of cardiovascular risk. He also stresses that a diet high in processed carbohydrates and sugars—not saturated fat—is the primary driver of dangerous cholesterol patterns. In his view, addressing underlying causes like insulin resistance, inflammation, and gut dysbiosis is key to truly improving heart health.

Mental Health: Get the Support You Deserve

The next step I always recommend is this: schedule an appointment with a licensed psychologist or mental health professional to get properly assessed. You may be dealing with PTSD, panic disorder, depression, or something else entirely—but knowing is the first step toward healing. Remember: you are in control of your health and your journey. Don't let anyone pressure you into treatments or approaches you're not comfortable with. Seek out second opinions when necessary, and talk to people you trust—friends, family, or mentors. You're not alone.

Start Where You Are

Whether you're just starting out or deep into your healing journey, take what resonates from this book and apply it to your life. Even small shifts can make a huge difference. Maybe one section stands out to you, start there. But don't stop there, branch out. There are so many amazing tools and perspectives out there. I personally benefited a lot from various courses on anxiety and panic, especially one focused on Cognitive Behavioral Therapy (CBT).

Physical Bodywork & Structural Support

It's not just about the mind and diet, but the body's structure plays a role too. I highly recommend getting an assessment from a qualified bodywork specialist, such as a craniosacral therapist, medical massage therapist, or structural integrator. These professionals can examine your spinal alignment, check for issues like scoliosis, and evaluate your upper cervical spine, including the atlas bone, which plays a major role in nervous system regulation. Don't overlook the tailbone (coccyx) either. Past injuries like falls can misalign it, creating discomfort, energetic blockages, or disruptions in the body's meridian and nervous system flow.

Taking care of these physical elements—just like nutrition and mental health—can be a crucial part of your full recovery or optimization. Every piece of the puzzle matters.

IMPORTANT NOTE:
There is growing evidence supporting the therapeutic use of psychoactive substances such as ketamine, psilocybin, and MDMA in professional treatment settings. Please do your own research, as I cannot provide any guidance here. What I can do is just bring awareness and encourage you to ask questions so you can make more informed decisions.

CAUTION: These therapies should only be explored under the guidance of qualified professionals at licensed treatment facilities and discussed directly with your mental health provider. This isn't just a disclaimer—it's a genuine safety consideration. Do your own research, approach with caution, and always prioritize your well-being.

Again, I want to be clear: I'm not against pharmaceuticals or psychiatric drug therapy when they're truly needed. But universally they're overprescribed. This has been talked about by so many professionals, doctors and experts in psychology and psychiatry. In many cases, especially during acute mental health crises, psychiatric medications can be lifesaving. For individuals struggling with severe anxiety, depression, or PTSD, medications like SSRIs or benzodiazepines (e.g., Xanax, Ativan, Klonopin) can offer real relief. They often work by altering brain chemistry—typically by increasing neurotransmitters like serotonin or GABA—to help reduce the intensity of symptoms.

That said, there are valid concerns about long-term use, especially when these medications are prescribed early in life or without a broader health plan. In children and teens, whose brains are still developing, prolonged use of anti-anxiety meds can sometimes blunt emotional development. Emotional flattening—where someone feels less anxious, but also disconnected, numb, or unmotivated—is a common experience reported by many users. This can delay the development of emotional resilience, self-regulation, and deeper healing.

For young adults, there's the added risk of becoming overly reliant on medication without addressing underlying root causes like trauma, nervous system dysregulation, poor lifestyle habits, or lack of emotional support. Benzodiazepines in particular carry a risk of tolerance and dependency, and abrupt withdrawal can trigger serious symptoms. Long-term use of some antidepressants has also been associated with side effects like sleep disruption, sexual dysfunction, weight gain, and increased suicidal thoughts in certain age groups.

However, let's be real—sometimes medication is exactly what someone needs to get through the day, reduce panic attacks, get sleep, or stabilize enough to start therapy. The key question is: *Are these medications being used as a short-term support tool while building real coping strategies, or are they becoming a permanent crutch?*

My message is not to shame or scare, but to advocate for informed, conscious decision making, especially for younger people. Medications have their place, but ideally, they should be part of a holistic healing plan that includes therapy, movement, proper nutrition, emotional support, and nervous system regulation. Without these, we risk masking symptoms instead of understanding them—and we miss the opportunity for true healing and long-term resilience.

What labs should you get?

Your doctor might be resistant to order some of these tests. I have NO IDEA why. Just tell them you've done some research along the lines of functional and naturopathic medicine for general health and chronic conditions. You don't need to do all these tests at once, I understand this might be overwhelming for you. I would try to do maybe half the tests and talk to your doctor about the ones that are most important. Minimally, you want to get all the standard testing and make sure you get *25 Hydroxy Vit D* and *fasting* Insulin. I highly recommend the NMR Lipid and CIMT tests if you think you might have plaque buildup due to your age and/or lifestyle. Tests that I recommend include:

- Complete metabolic panel
- CBC Complete blood count
- UA Urinalysis
- Fractionated Lipid NMR Panel, a highly detailed and advanced Cholesterol Lipid test. You might have to pay for this one ($100–$150), but it's worth it to do at least two in a row to find out where you are.
- CIMT Test – Carotid Intima–Media Thickness – testing the carotid artery of any plaque buildup. (It's been proven that atherosclerosis, the plaque buildup in the arteries has and can be healed FULLY—Dr. Stephen Hussey talks about this.)
- CAC Score – Coronary Artery Calcium – sees the plaque buildup around the heart. Score of ZERO is what you're after. This is a CAT scan so if you have to choose, decide with your doctor, but do the CIMT ultrasound first, to possibly avoid the CAT scan radiation.
- Fasting Insulin – optimal is 5 or less. 7 is safe range.
- Vitamin D 25 Hydroxy – optimal is 50–70. Some have more,

some with very high scores (over 80) may have issues with the immune dysfunction but this doesn't apply to everyone.
- A1c – shows whether you're pre–diabetic. Over 5.7 – you may have what's known as 'dawn phenomenon.' The dawn phenomenon is a natural rise in blood sugar levels that happens in the early morning, usually between 2 a.m. and 8 a.m. This occurs because the body releases hormones like cortisol, adrenaline, and growth hormone to prepare you for waking up. These hormones signal the liver to release glucose (sugar) into the bloodstream for energy.

  In most people, insulin balances this out—but in those with insulin resistance, prediabetes, or diabetes, blood sugar can spike too high upon waking. It's not caused by eating late at night, but by your body's internal clock and hormone rhythms. Managing stress, sleep, and evening meals can help reduce its effect. Insulin resistance might be what you are having, like I had.
- Homa – IR – Insulin resistance test
- Oral Glucose Tolerance test – checks the health of you Insulin response
- **Testosterone levels and optimal ranges**: This section mainly applies to men because anxiety and depression in men are often linked to low testosterone levels. In contrast, women rarely experience problems from low testosterone—indeed, higher levels of testosterone in women tend to reduce anxiety and stress, although they can be other health concerns beyond the scope of this book. Men, on the other hand, seldom struggle with excessively high testosterone; their primary hormonal risk comes from having too little. Maintaining testosterone in an optimal range is therefore especially important for men's mental well–being.

  Testosterone levels naturally vary by age, but standard reference ranges for men are:
    - Ages 19 to 49: **249 – 836 ng/dL**
    - Ages 50 and older: **193 – 740 ng/dL**

However, these are general clinical ranges, not necessarily optimal ones. In my experience and research, **men over 40 should aim for levels of at least 400 ng/dL**, with **500 ng/dL with higher being more ideal**. A reading in the low 300s for a man over 40 is often considered suboptimal, even if it technically falls within the "normal" range.

Speaking as someone who had low testosterone in early adulthood, I can say the difference in how you feel is profound. Optimizing testosterone takes effort, it doesn't just happen on its own. But it's well worth it. As discussed in the previous chapter, testosterone plays a vital role not just in physical health (like muscle mass, energy, and libido), but also in **mental and emotional well-being**. It's closely linked to resilience against **chronic conditions, anxiety, depression, and mood disorders**.

- B vitamins, especially B6 B9 and B12
- Thyroid – these tests should give you a solid view of your thyroid
    - TSH
    - Free T3 and T4
    - Reverse T3
    - Thyroglobulin Antibodies TGAB
- Genetic Testing
    - SOD2 SNP
    - NQO1 (Coq10 Problems)
- Immune System Tests
    - TH1/TH2 Cytokine profile (IL–2, IL–4, IL10, TNF–Alpha)
    - Immunoglobulin Panel (IgG+ subclasses, IgA, IgM, IgE)
    - CD4/CD8 T–cell ratios
    - Viral reactivation panels (Epstein Barr, CMV cytomegalovirus, HHV–6 / HSV Herpes) Chronic Viral infections can contribute to immune system dysregulation, chronic conditions and anxiety driven physical sensations.

- Antinuclear Antibody test (ANA) – this test can identify possible autoimmune conditions and even leaky gut.
- Homocysteine Levels
  - MTHFR
  - MTRR
  - MTR
  - COMT
  - FUT2

Note on Uric Acid and Low–Carb Diets

Uric acid is a natural waste product formed from the breakdown of purines, which are found in many foods—especially meat, seafood, and alcohol. While the standard laboratory reference range for uric acid is typically 3.5 to 7.2 mg/dL in people, optimal levels are generally considered to be below 5.5 mg/dL, particularly when assessing long–term metabolic and cardiovascular health. In my research and experience, if you follow a strict low–carb or carnivore/ketogenic diet for an extended period, your uric acid levels may temporarily rise to 6–7 mg/dL or slightly higher. This can happen during the initial stages of ketosis due to increased breakdown of purines and changes in kidney excretion. However, this does not automatically indicate a problem (such as gout), especially if you're not experiencing symptoms like joint pain or swelling.

On the other hand, if you follow a standard high–carbohydrate diet and your uric acid levels are consistently above 6.5 or 7 mg/dL, this may be a warning sign. Elevated uric acid in that context has been associated with increased risk of gout, insulin resistance, metabolic syndrome, and cardiovascular issues. In such cases, dietary and lifestyle adjustments may be necessary. Always consult a qualified healthcare provider for interpretation of lab results in context, especially if you have other risk factors or symptoms.

Takeaways from Chapter 4

- Go to the doctor.
- Don't hesitate to get basic blood work, physical exams, and screenings. Even simple tests can bring peace of mind and direction.
- Find a psychologist you feel comfortable with. A solid therapeutic relationship can provide a safe space for healing, growth, and emotional processing.
- Take time to reflect, consider, and evaluate whether psychiatric support could be helpful. If you feel it may be, consult with a professional who aligns with your values, especially if you prefer a more natural and minimal approach to medication.
- When speaking with any healthcare professional, express your preferences clearly. Remember, you are a unique individual, not just a set of symptoms.
- Open up to a trusted loved one. Talking things through with someone close to you can be incredibly grounding. Ask for their thoughts and support.
- See a bodywork professional. Explore options like craniosacral therapy, medical massage, or chiropractic care. **Just a side note, I personally don't like chiropractors twisting and popping my neck. Don't feel bad about letting them know not to do that if you see them.** Structural imbalances in the body can impact mental health more than we often realize.
- Reconsider what you've been told about cholesterol. Cholesterol isn't the villain we were led to believe it is. Understand the underlying metabolic and inflammatory factors that matter more.
- Diagnosis or no diagnosis—both paths have value.

- A diagnosis can provide clarity, direction, and a sense of relief. But not having one can be equally valuable; it means you've ruled things out and can keep moving forward with greater focus.
- Healing is still possible, even without a clear label.

Chapter 5
Signs, Symptoms and Sensations of Panic and Anxiety

"Being able to feel safe with other people is probably the single most important aspect of mental health; Safe connections are fundamental to having meaningful and satisfying lives."
— Bessel Van Der Kolk

Panic is often just the body and mind *thinking* or *perceiving* that you're in danger even when you're not. In those moments, try asking yourself: *"Am I actually in danger right now, or is this just an irrational fear that my body is reacting to?"* That one question alone can start to shift your perspective.

Most of the time, the answer will be obvious: *"No, I'm not in real danger."* You might be lying in bed, walking into a store, or driving down the road when out of nowhere, irrational thoughts pop up— doom and gloom, worst–case scenarios, the never–ending stream of *"what if?"* questions.

These thoughts can quickly cause your mind to spiral. If they gain momentum, they can build into full–blown anxiety or even panic. That spiral is real, and it can feel overwhelming. But sometimes, simply recognizing what's happening and stepping in to rationalize with your own thoughts can start to break the cycle. This is one of the key tools to help manage panic and anxiety. By the way—if you haven't noticed yet, colors play a subtle but powerful role in how we feel. Blue is often associated with calm and serenity, especially lighter shades. Green, tied to nature, tends to create a sense of balance and harmony. Little things like this matter more than we realize.

Don't forget: **Anxiety is a normal human experience.** If you're about to speak in front of an audience, go to a big interview, or perform in any way, it's completely natural to feel nervous or even anxious. That's good stress; it means you care, and it can actually help you focus and perform better. But the problem starts when your mind catastrophizes—imagining extreme, irrational scenarios. That's when anxiety stops being useful and starts taking over. If left unchecked, that mental spiral is what can trigger panic. The goal is to learn to recognize those thought patterns *before* they escalate. From there, you can bring yourself back into the moment, calm your nervous system, and take back control.

Common symptoms of panic and anxiety include:
- Having a sense of impending danger, panic or doom
- Fear of loss of control or death
- Rapid, pounding heart rate
- Sweating or chills
- Trembling or shaking
- Shortness of breath or tightness in your throat
- Hot flashes
- Nausea
- Abdominal cramping
- Chest pain
- Headache
- Dizziness, lightheadedness or faintness
- Numbness or tingling sensation
- Feeling of unreality or detachment
- Feeling nervous, restless or tense
- Breathing rapidly (hyperventilation)
- Feeling weak or tired
- Trouble concentrating or thinking about anything other than the present worry
- Having trouble sleeping
- Experiencing gastrointestinal (GI) problems
- Having the urge to avoid things that trigger anxiety
- Constant swallowing/lump in the throat.

If you're experiencing technical difficulties in the mental or emotional realm—like an anxiety or panic attack—try finding quick relief through a guided EFT (Emotional Freedom Technique) session. This is something I used which helped me immensely. I recommend searching YouTube for a follow-along video by Brad Yates. His sessions are simple, calming, and surprisingly effective for many people.

This is also why I encourage you to see a doctor to get a full physical. Ask for comprehensive blood work, metabolic panels, hormone testing, and food or allergy sensitivity testing. Make sure you have a clear picture of what's going on in your body. And don't hesitate to ask your doctor what *they* recommend as well, you might uncover something valuable you hadn't thought of.

If you're dealing with chronic illness, autoimmune symptoms, or unexplained fatigue, it's crucial that you bring those up. Getting answers helped bring peace of mind and gave me more confidence moving forward. We've come a long way in dealing with chronic illness in the past 20 years. There's so much help and support out there, including this book and the doctors and experts I've researched. Many of them specialize in chronic illness and a lot of the "unexplained symptoms" that has the average doctor so confused.

The point is: it's important to know what you're working with. When you find out that your body is physically healthy—or at least understand what's going on—you can begin to rule out some of the possible causes behind your symptoms, triggers, and anxieties. That clarity helps you move forward with a sense of direction, rather than being stuck in fear or confusion.

When someone is experiencing PTSD, panic, or hyperventilation, the nervous system can feel intensely "buzzy"—like a low-grade electrical current running through the body. This sensation often stems from the sympathetic nervous system being stuck in overdrive—what we know as the fight-or-flight state. With PTSD, the brain becomes hypervigilant, constantly scanning for danger even when there's no threat. Hyperventilation—rapid, shallow breathing—throws off the balance between oxygen and carbon dioxide, disrupting the body's pH levels and triggering a cascade of adrenaline and nervous energy. The result? That buzzing, jittery, restless, shaky, or even tingling feeling. It's the body's way of saying, "I'm overwhelmed and bracing for impact."

IMPORTANT NOTE
What you're feeling is your body trying to protect you. It's not a sign that you're broken. With the right tools, support, and mindset, you can teach your system to feel safe again.

Have you ever wondered about the difference between panic and anxiety? The short version: anxiety is a more manageable, lower-level version of panic. Panic is what happens when anxiety spirals out of control—usually triggered by catastrophizing thoughts and irrational "what if" scenarios that build on each other until the body reacts intensely.

It's also important to check in with your body and symptoms. If you're running a fever, have body aches, or a cough—it's probably not anxiety. Especially in the age of COVID-19, many people have heightened health anxiety, unsure whether their sensations are physical illness or emotional overwhelm.

Something that doesn't get talked about enough are the symptoms that come before and after a high-anxiety or panic episode. Beforehand, it often starts with that creeping anxious feeling. Your thoughts become scattered, irrational, distorted. (We'll break down these distortions later on.) Mild physical symptoms can also start to surface—tight chest, shaky hands, stomach upset. It's usually that simple.

After a panic episode, you might feel shaken, confused, or even scared by what just happened. Many people feel wiped out—it takes a lot of energy to go through that state. If it was brief, maybe you bounce back quickly. But if you've been in a state of prolonged anxiety or stress, it can leave you completely drained. You may also feel light-headed, spacey, or disassociated. Digestive issues can linger as well. Personally, even though it's generally not great to eat while you're stressed, I felt eating comforted me in times of high anxiety and panic situations. That's why they call carbohydrates and grains comfort foods.

But keep in mind that this isn't a sustainable eating habit! It was just a way back then years ago now, to be able to help bring the fire down and get me to the next step. This is a big problem with a lot of people. This one thing, stress eating, contributes to obesity rates and other health problems that we spoke about in previous chapters. The idea is to get to a point where you're ideally grain free for a while and to heal the gut microbiome and fix nutrient deficiencies.

I don't love using labels, but I want to explain something: the term "anxiety/panic disorder" often applies when someone begins to fear the fear itself. You become afraid of the idea of having another panic attack, and that fear leads you to avoid certain places, activities, or people. That's exactly where I was—and why I'm writing this book now. Because I've been there, and no human should have to live in that kind of fear.

Sometimes, anxiety is your body's way of nudging you to look inward. Maybe there is a rational message underneath it all—a lesson, a signal, or an invitation to grow. This journey isn't just about escaping anxiety; it's about learning from it. We'll unpack more of that in the coming sections.

Lastly, I want to acknowledge something real: most people cope with anxiety and stress through substances—alcohol, cigarettes, drugs. For centuries, that's been the cultural go-to. But this book is here to show you another way. A healthier, more sustainable way to manage stress, anxiety, and PTSD—without self-destruction or addiction.

IMPORTANT NOTE:
You need to know that you're not entirely at the mercy of anxiety and panic. While it's true that your autonomic nervous system operates mostly beneath your conscious control, you can influence it, and that's a major focus of this book. Through specific techniques like breathwork, cognitive behavioral tools, EFT, mindset shifts, and other nervous system exercises, you'll learn how to interrupt the cycle of fear, restore balance, and invite more calm and resilience into your daily life.

Attachment Styles

Learning about attachment styles were an important part of my healing and understanding of my C–PTSD. **What are attachment styles?** Founded by psychoanalyst John Bowlby in the 1950s and expanded by Mary Ainsworth, attachment theory outlines how your bond with your primary caregivers sets the foundation for how you navigate relationships throughout life. I highly recommend reading a book on this.

The four attachment styles are:
- Secure – (safe and stable)
- Avoidant – (dismissive, or anxious–avoidant in children)
- Anxious – (preoccupied, or anxious–ambivalent in children)
- Disorganized – (fearful–avoidant in children)

Secure attachment style is characterized by the ability to build strong secure lasting relationships in your life. Ultimately, you felt safe, understood, comforted, and valued during your early interactions. Your caregivers were emotionally stable.

Signs of a secure attachment style include:
- Ability to regulate your emotions
- Easily trusting others
- Effective communication skills
- Ability to seek emotional support

- Comfortable being alone and in close relationships
- Ability to self-reflect in partnerships
- Being easy to connect with
- Ability to manage conflict well
- High self-esteem
- Ability to be emotionally available

Secure attachment people form healthy relationships with others, have less negative emotions, and can engage in the world in a healthy way. Basically, it's the style we're all after!

Anxious attachment style is characterized by fear and abandonment, codependent tendencies, and looking for validation and emotional regulation from others.

Signs you might have an anxious attachment style include:
- Clingy tendencies
- Highly sensitive to criticism (real or perceived)
- Needing approval from others
- Jealous tendencies
- Difficulty being alone
- Low self-esteem
- Feeling unworthy of love
- Intense fear of rejection
- Significant fear of abandonment
- Difficulty trusting others

If you have an anxious attachment style, your parents may have also had:
- Alternated between being overly coddling and detached or indifferent
- Been easily overwhelmed
- Been sometimes attentive and then push you away
- Made you responsible for how they felt

In relationships you may be the one trying to take care of others but are also codependent and needy. You may feel unworthy of love and require consistent reassurance. You might blame yourself for challenges in the relationship and experience jealousy due to low self-esteem. There might be a deep-rooted fear of abandonment, loneliness or a feeling of rejection, which are often at the root of relationship issues, codependency and the other feelings listed above.

Avoidant attachment style is characterized by insecurity. Basically, you don't allow yourself to get very close emotionally and physically in relationships for fear of being hurt. In your childhood, you might have had strict or emotionally distant and absent caregivers.

Your parents or caregivers might have:
- Left you to fend for yourself
- Expected you to be independent
- Been slow to respond to your basic needs
- Reprimanded you for depending on them
- Rejected you when expressing your needs or emotions

Some parents can be neglectful, or even just busy, disinterested and focused more on rational things in life like grades, chores and getting things done. Therefore, some people grow up with a sense of independence and they might want to always depend on themselves rather than others. This will manifest in keeping their distance from others and intimate partners.

You might have an anxious-avoidant attachment style if you:
- Persistently avoid emotional or physical intimacy
- Feel a strong sense of independence
- Are uncomfortable expressing your feelings
- Are dismissive of others
- Have a hard time trusting people.
- Feel threatened by anyone who tries to get close to you
- Spend more time alone than interacting with others
- Believe you don't need others in your life.
- Have commitment issues

These people may engage in relationships, but they avoid getting close emotionally. A partner might feel as if they can't get inside and will inevitably be pushed away or dismissed when the relationship feels too serious for the anxious–avoidant partner.

Disorganized attachment style is characterized by very inconsistent behavior and a difficult time trusting others. This style forms from childhood trauma, abuse or neglect. Fear of caregivers can also be seen. Caregivers are inconsistent and they may provide comfort one minute, but cause fear the next, which creates confusion in the child.

Signs of a disorganized attachment style include:
- Difficulty trusting others
- Fear of rejection
- Inability to regulate emotions
- Contradictory behaviors
- High levels of anxiety

Having both an anxious and avoidant attachment style

Some mental health concerns stem from this type of attachment style, including mood disorders, personality disorders, self–harm, or substance use disorders. These types are all over the place, they want intimacy but then push away. They confuse others and are confused themselves. They might be independent and then clingy and emotional, ultimately wrestling with wanting security and the fear that arises. Others may see them as a really intense person and they can become tense in their bodies because of it. People with this attachment stye often rely on escapism by constantly staying busy. This then often fuels the addiction to working and staying busy, often along with drug and alcohol abuse.

Becoming "a doer" often happens in childhood. Achieving and doing good overall are common coping strategies for children when they might feel unsafe and/or are in a chaotic environment. This can also happen in a home where the parents are doers. These types of parents push the kids to do a laundry list of schooling and recreational activities. This also applies to authoritarian, religious or military style households.

This often leads to a child who constantly tries to win the parent over, so they don't get mad or upset at them. As they grow up, they might work so hard to get away from a broken home. They may struggle with intimacy. Doers tend not to process feeling and emotions and just go straight to fix everything by doing it. Others need to chase them to connect.

What are trauma personalities?

These are personality types that are developed from a traumatic childhood, which are not our true authentic personalities. Patrick Teahan talks about five of them. I highly recommend watching his videos and content. Trauma personalities stem from the idea that our traumas and troubled childhoods put us in a negative emotional state that snowballs into personality dysfunction. We're all born with a divine spark (in my personal opinion) and many professionals and experts would agree. But this divinity and innocence gets distorted, skewed and suffocated by negative emotions such as anger, sadness, fear, loneliness, disappointment or jealousy. This does not mean a child can't become more mature at a young age and take more responsibility and live a successful life!

Trauma personalities are really rooted in fight, flight, freeze, shutdown, shame, submit, and cry for help. Let's go over some basic information on what kinds of personality issues we can have as adults that stem from childhood trauma.

- **Emotional dysregulation** – difficulty managing emotions and feeling of intense anger, sadness, anxiety, angst, fear, usually without clear triggers.
- **Trust issues** – problems trusting others because of past abuse and trauma coming from others.

- **Low self–esteem** – feelings of worthlessness or inadequacy, which can stem from negative self–perceptions during traumatic experiences.
- **Fear of abandonment** – intense fear of being abandoned or rejected which can lead to clingy needy behavior, preemptively pushing others away.
- **Hypervigilance** – constant state of alertness or readiness for danger, triggering more anxiety and or panic.
- **Dissociation** – frequent episodes of dissociation where individuals feel detached from themselves and surroundings. This will affect their ability to stay present, which in turn affects focus concentration, school, relationships, jobs or career.
- **Difficulty with boundaries** – either being too rigid and stubborn, or too permissive and allowing others to take advantage.
- **Chronic feelings with emptiness** – becoming apathetic, numb and feeling like there is a void, which can lead to self-destructive, addictive behavior and/or constant seeking of external validation.
- **Negative self-perception** – internalized negative belief about oneself stemming from abusive experiences during childhood.
- **Difficulty with intimacy** – fear of vulnerability from past trauma.
- **Persistent guilt and shame** – chronic feelings of guilt and shame coming from traumatic experiences that often leads to the belief that you are somehow to blame.
- **Perfectionism** – a drive to be perfect as a way to cope with feelings of inadequacy or to avoid criticism and rejection.
- **Avoidant behavior** – tendency to avoid situations, people or emotions that might bring up or trigger traumatic memories or feelings of vulnerability.

These are the kinds of things that can be very helpful to talk to a health professional about. You might find that by talking things out and getting helpful feedback, you might just not be at fault for something you've been carrying for years. You may end up understanding why you might be trying to be perfect all the time and why you think that if you're not then there's something "wrong" with you.

The Nervous System

The nervous system consists of the central nervous system (CNS) and the peripheral nervous system (PNS). The nervous system plays a big part in the body's reaction and response to stress, anxiety and panic. Understanding the anatomy and function will help you understand what's happening in your body and how it plays out in your mind.

The CNS consists of the brain and spinal cord. The PNS is the part that branches out from the brain and spinal cord to the rest of the body and communicates with the central nervous system, aka the brain. The PNS has two parts to it. The autonomic and somatic nervous system. The autonomic nervous system regulates the involuntary physiologic processes, including heart rate, blood pressure, respiration, digestion, sexual arousal, and the important fight, flight or freeze response. Your somatic nervous system is a subdivision of your peripheral nervous system that stretches throughout nearly every part of your body. The nerves in this system deliver information from your senses to your brain. They also carry commands from your brain to your muscles so you can move around.

The two branches of the autonomic nervous system deserve a closer look:

Sympathetic Nervous System

Often called the "fight, flight, or freeze" system, the sympathetic nervous system gears us up for action. It increases heart rate, raises blood pressure, triggers sweating, and floods the body with adrenaline—everything we need to meet a challenge or escape danger.

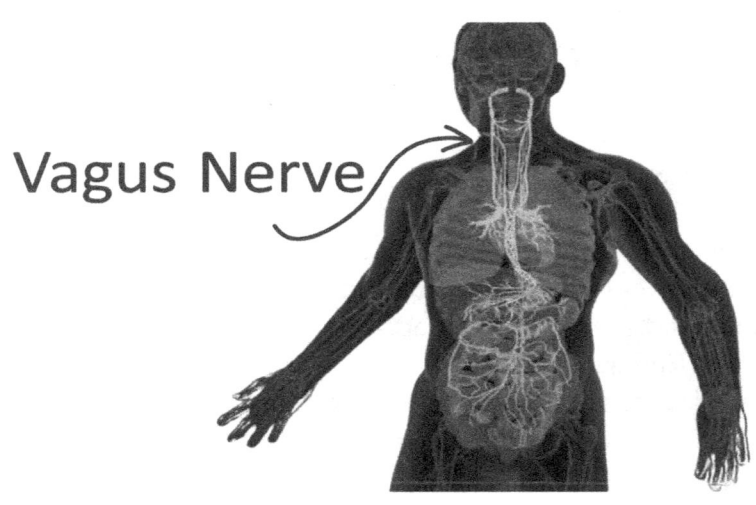

In Taoist and Qigong terms, this is Yang energy: active, outward, and masculine.

Parasympathetic Nervous System

In contrast, the parasympathetic system (sometimes called "rest and digest") brings us back to center. It slows the heart, promotes digestion, supports recovery, and readies us for sleep. This is the Yin side—calming, inward, and feminine—and it's essential for restoring balance after sympathetic activation.

When life's demands or past traumas push us into a persistent state of stress, we can become sympathetic–dominant. In this mode, our bodies lose resilience: we're stuck in high–alert, and the parasympathetic "brakes" struggle to engage. Over time, that chronic activation undermines health, making it harder to recover from everyday stresses or traumatic triggers. Understanding—and learning to shift between—these two systems is a key step toward regaining your natural balance.

Next, we'll talk about the vagus nerve which is part of the "Parasympathetic" nervous system.

The vagus nerve, also known as the 10th cranial nerve, is one of the longest nerves in the body and plays a vital role in the parasympathetic nervous system. This nerve is one of the most important nerves in the body, if not the most important when it comes to PTSD, anxiety and panic disorders, chronic illnesses and of course homeostasis (internal stability). This system regulates various involuntary bodily functions and organs, including digestion, heart rate, immune response, breathing, lungs, heart, and adrenal glands.

When an individual experiences stress that their body struggles to alleviate, they remain in a heightened state of sympathetic dominance. While this heightened state can initially provide a surge of energy, it often leads to a decline in digestive function, restless sleep, and morning fatigue. Over time, this persistent stress response can lead to adrenal exhaustion, commonly known as burnout.

Here are a few signs that your vagus nerve might need attention:
- PTSD/ C–PTSD
- Anxiety and/panic attacks
- Feelings of disconnection to your environment
- Sensory sensitivity (to lights, sounds, touch)
- Emotional numbness – apathy
- Gut/ digestive issues (gas, bloating, IBS, irritation of digestion)
- Hypervigilance and being constantly on edge, even paranoid
- Frequent dissociation
- Insomnia
- Feeling tired but wired
- Feeling helpless, hopeless or stuck
- Abdominal pain and bloating
- Acid reflux (gastroesophageal reflux disease, GERD)
- Changes to heart rate, blood pressure or blood sugar
- Difficulty swallowing or loss of gag reflex
- Dizziness or fainting
- Hoarseness, wheezing or loss of voice

Vagus Nerve Techniques, Tips and Tricks

Vagus nerve stimulation can be a gentle, safe, and powerful tool for supporting recovery from trauma, PTSD, chronic pain, anxiety, and more. That said, like with any practice, it's important to proceed with all the information and care. If you have bradycardia (a persistently slow heart rate) or brady–tachycardia (an uncommon condition in which your heart rhythm cycles between slow and fast), please approach vagus–nerve exercises with extra caution. In my own experience with brady–tachycardia, I was able to benefit from gentle techniques—light massage and soothing breathing exercises—only during moments when I felt stable or mildly anxious. Over time, as my nervous system found its balance, this condition resolved.

It's also worth noting that well–trained athletes often have naturally lower resting heart rates than the general population. In my case, repeated "freeze" responses due to trauma contributed to a chronically dysregulated nervous system and the associated heart–rate fluctuations. With mindful practice and proper guidance, however, vagal–tone exercises can still support recovery—so long as you **listen to your body** and move at a pace that feels safe and manageable. Go slow, and consult with a qualified healthcare professional if you're unsure. When used appropriately, these exercises can be a valuable and empowering part of your healing toolkit.

By keeping these precautions in mind, you can safely incorporate vagus nerve exercises into your routine. These first techniques I will share are the ones I've used personally and have found helpful.

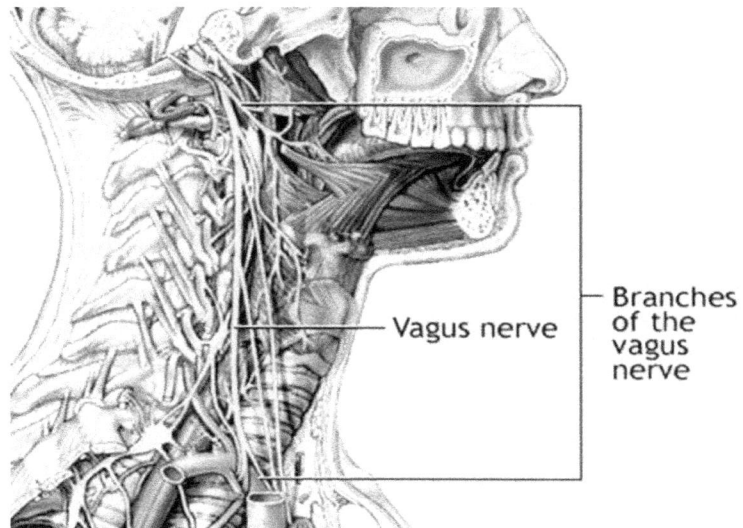

Vagus nerve

Branches of the vagus nerve

Ear Massage

The vagus nerve runs in and around the ears as it travels down the side of the neck and into the body. In the evening time, I would simply massage all around my ears, the outside, the inside (concha), behind the ears on the skull and on the tragus (the pointed cartilage just outside the ear canal) is also important. You want your ears to move around loosely and be relaxed. You'll probably find that your ears are full of tensions and crackles in the cartilage. Spend a minute or two before bed or anytime you're feeling anxious or stressed.

Neck Massage

> **IMPORTANT NOTE:**
> **Avoid massaging the carotid artery area (the sides of the neck) in older adults or in anyone with suspected atherosclerosis, arterial plaque, cardiovascular disease, or hardening of the arteries. Stimulating this area could increase the risk of dislodging plaque, which may lead to stroke or heart attack.**

Carotid sinus massage is a simple technique that stimulates the vagus nerve by gently massaging the area of the neck where the carotid artery splits, just below the jawline. This can help activate the parasympathetic nervous system, which slows the heart rate and promotes a state of calm and relaxation. It's sometimes used clinically to manage certain types of rapid heart rate. However, it should be done gently and with caution, especially in older adults or those with cardiovascular issues, and ideally under guidance, as applying pressure to the carotid artery can affect blood flow and displace arterial plaque. When done safely and one side at a time, it can be a useful tool to help calm anxiety, reduce stress, and support vagus nerve activation. You can simply take your fingers and massage down the sides of the neck with circles or just slowly swiping straight down. It takes a couple minutes to do this.

Diaphragmatic Breathing/Balloon Breathing

This way of breathing is a powerful way to activate the vagus nerve and calm the nervous system. In this practice, you breathe deeply into your belly, like inflating a balloon, allowing the diaphragm to fully expand and contract. This gentle, rhythmic movement stimulates the vagus nerve, which runs through the diaphragm and signals the body to shift out of fight–or–flight mode and into rest–and–digest. As you slow the breath and extend your exhale, the vagus nerve tells the brain that you are safe, which reduces the heart rate, lowers cortisol, and brings a sense of calm and groundedness. This technique is especially helpful for managing anxiety, emotional overwhelm, and nervous system dysregulation.

Cold Water/ Cold Therapy

Cold sensation activates the vagal tone. For most of my life, I would stand up from sitting or lying down, get up to go to the bathroom and while standing there, my heart would be pounding and start racing (POTS – tachycardia – dysautonomia symptoms) and I would have to cut myself off and run to the sink and splash cold water on my face and it would help immediately. You can also try putting cold packs from the freezer on one side of the neck for 15 to 20 seconds and then switching sides a few times.

Gargling water, Gagging, Humming or Singing

Laryngeal/pharyngeal nerves that are branches of the vagus nerve, extend into the throat. This is why gargling and the gagging reflex helps to activate the vagus nerve. Use the toothbrush to gag yourself at night before bed and then gargle after brushing. Humming and singing will activate the vagus nerve.

Bearing Down: The Valsalva maneuver

Bearing down means that you try to breathe out with your stomach muscles, but you don't let air out of your nose or mouth. You can do this while blowing on the tip of your thumb in your mouth. Basically, holding your breath while pretending to push like you're going to the bathroom. This is the typical version of the Valsalva Maneuver.

The Modified Valsalva Maneuver is where you sit and take a breath in and hold and bear down for 15 seconds. Don't bear down too much so that it creates pressure in the head. After 15 seconds, lay flat and raise legs 45 degrees for 15 seconds. The legs should be passive, propped up on something or having someone hold them up. Return to seated and relax. This is also used for supra ventricular tachycardia (SVT) and arrhythmias. Afterwards it may take up to a minute or so for you to return to normal.

PANIC TO POTENTIAL TOOL:
There are videos on YouTube about these exercises and the Valsalva Maneuver, which will be helpful to watch.

Eye Massage and Movements

Gently massaging around the eyes and practicing slow, intentional eye movements, especially looking left and right, can help stimulate the vagus nerve and calm the nervous system. The vagus nerve is connected to the ocular muscles and areas around the face through the brainstem, and engaging the eyes in this way taps into the body's natural calming pathways. Light circular massage around the eye sockets, combined with soft, side–to–side eye tracking (without moving the head), can signal safety to the brain, reduce stored tension, and bring the body into a more relaxed, parasympathetic state. This technique is subtle yet powerful, especially for those managing anxiety, trauma, or nervous system imbalances.

Exercise

Hormones released during relaxing or moderate exercise help activate the vagus nerve. Do things like calisthenics, yoga, qigong, Pilates, meditation, light activities, dancing, or swimming, find what you enjoy!

Connecting with Others and Laughter

Finding a sense of community, having good company, laughing and having a good time, all help your vagal tone.

Visualizations

Visualizations actually help regulate the vagus nerve. Think back to a time when life felt easier and your mind was at peace. Picture that moment clearly—whether it really happened or it's a comforting scene you create in your imagination. Use it like a simple meditation: bring yourself there, notice the sights and sounds, and let that calm, worry–free feeling settle in your body.

Neuroception

This is a term coined by Dr. Stephen Porges, the creator of the Polyvagal Theory, to describe the subconscious process our nervous system uses to detect safety, danger, or life–threatening situations in our environment. Unlike perception, which involves conscious awareness, neuroception happens automatically, without our control, as part of the autonomic nervous system's role in keeping us safe. It's a key factor in how we react to stress and trauma, including PTSD.

Neuroception is constantly scanning for cues of safety or danger. It assesses external factors (like facial expressions, body language, or tone of voice) and internal factors (such as bodily sensations or memories) to determine whether we are safe, at risk, or in immediate danger. Based on these assessments, it triggers different responses through the autonomic nervous system:

- **Safety:** When the environment feels safe, the parasympathetic nervous system (via the vagus nerve) helps us feel calm, connected, and social.
- **Danger:** If neuroception detects danger, the sympathetic nervous system kicks in, preparing us for "fight or flight" by increasing heart rate, adrenaline, and alertness.
- **Life–threatening:** In extreme cases, when the threat feels overwhelming or inescapable, the dorsal vagal complex (another part of the parasympathetic nervous system) may activate, causing a "freeze" response, where the body shuts down to protect itself.

In individuals with PTSD, neuroception can become dysregulated. Trauma alters the nervous system, making it hypersensitive to perceived threats—even in situations where there may be no real danger. This heightened state of vigilance can lead to:

Hyperarousal: The nervous system stays stuck in a constant state of alert, causing symptoms like anxiety, insomnia, and irritability. I've had this myself and seen this very often in the healing and yoga community, where the person goes to a healing retreat or does lots of therapy and their nervous system is humming or buzzing, which can feel very uncomfortable. Not to mention they are probably too low in nutrients, particularly vitamin B1 and other vitamins. This happens because they start to open up the can of worms so to speak, trauma and PTSD experiences and they become dysregulated in the process. They need the techniques from this book to find homeostasis.

Hypervigilance: Individuals may continuously scan their environment for threats, feeling on edge and unable to relax.

Overactive Fight or Flight Responses: Even mild stressors can trigger exaggerated physiological responses, such as a racing heart, sweating, or shallow breathing.

Freeze Response: Some PTSD sufferers may experience dissociation or numbness as part of the freeze response, where the brain shuts down to avoid overwhelming emotional or physical pain.

When neuroception is out of balance, the brain can mistake neutral or safe situations for dangerous ones, keeping the body locked in survival mode. For someone with PTSD, this can lead to constant feelings of fear, anxiety, and emotional exhaustion. Everyday events, like a loud noise or a certain smell, can trigger intense memories of trauma because the nervous system interprets them as threats, even when the conscious mind knows otherwise.

Over time, this chronic stress can lead to physical issues like gastrointestinal problems, heart disease, and weakened immune function. The body isn't designed to stay in a perpetual state of fight, flight, or freeze.

IMPORTANT NOTE:
There are devices out there now that are vagus nerve stimulators and other wearable devices that you wear on your wrist or ankle and other places, which vibrate and bring calm and peace to the body and mind, including the:

Apollo Neuro, a wearable that sends gentle vibrations to your nervous system to calm the nervous system, the whole body and mind. My wife wears this one and she loves it.

Pulsetto, a vagus nerve stimulator that you wear around the neck and that sends stimulation directly to the vagus nerves in the neck.

VerRelief, another vagus nerve stimulator that has handheld and headphone options. My wife also has one of these and it has been very helpful. For the last part of this chapter, let's define a couple important things and look further into PTSD and anxiety.

What is the difference between feelings and emotions?

Though often used interchangeably, emotions and feelings are distinct concepts, each playing a different role in how we experience and interpret the world around us. Understanding the difference between the two can help you better navigate your internal experiences and gain insight into how your mind and body work together.

Emotions are the body's immediate, automatic responses to stimuli. They arise from the unconscious parts of the brain, particularly the limbic system. The primary limbic system function is to process and regulate emotion and memory while also dealing with sexual stimulation and learning. Behavior and the HPA axis is also interconnected with this and are closely linked to physiological reactions in the body. Emotions are often triggered without conscious thought and are part of our evolutionary survival mechanism, helping us quickly respond to threats, opportunities, and challenges.

Emotions are hardwired into our biology and serve as a fundamental survival tool. For example, fear triggers the fight–or–flight–or–freeze response, which prepares the body to deal with danger. Emotions occur quickly and tend to be brief, lasting anywhere from a few seconds to minutes. Basic emotions like joy, anger, fear, sadness, and disgust are universal across human cultures and even across species. Emotions cause physical reactions, such as increased heart rate, sweating, or changes in facial expressions (e.g., smiling when happy, frowning when sad).

Feelings, on the other hand, are the conscious, subjective interpretations of those emotions. While emotions are automatic and arise from unconscious brain processes, feelings are the result of conscious thought. They are influenced by personal experiences, beliefs, memories, and context. In other words, feelings are the way we make sense of and label our emotions.

Feelings involve a mental process where we interpret and label our emotional experiences. For instance, the emotion of fear might lead to a feeling of anxiety or insecurity, depending on the context. Feelings tend to linger longer than emotions. While an emotional reaction might pass quickly, the feeling it generates can last for hours, days, or even longer.

Unlike emotions, which are universal, feelings are highly personal and shaped by individual experiences, culture, and background. Two people might experience the same emotion but interpret and feel it differently. Feelings can be mixed and more nuanced than basic emotions. For example, you might feel bittersweet about a change in life, experiencing a combination of sadness and excitement.

Consider the emotion of fear and the feeling of anxiety. Fear is an immediate, primal response to a perceived threat. When you encounter danger, your body reacts with fear to help protect you— your heart rate increases, adrenaline floods your system, and you become more alert. Once the threat passes, the emotion of fear subsides.

Anxiety is the feeling that often follows the emotion of fear. It's the conscious interpretation of your body's response, and it might linger even after the danger has passed. You may continue to feel anxious or uneasy for a while, as your mind processes what happened and contemplates potential future threats. Anxiety can be tied to fear, but it's more about your subjective experience and thoughts surrounding that emotion.

Emotions and feelings are closely linked but operate in a sequence: emotions come first, followed by feelings. When you experience an emotional reaction, your brain processes the physical changes in your body (heart rate, sweating, wellbeing, facial expressions) and uses past experiences, memories, and context to interpret what that emotion means. This interpretation becomes your feeling.

For example, you see a snake (stimulus), and your body automatically responds with fear (emotion) as your heart races and adrenaline kicks in. Afterward, your mind processes the experience, and you might interpret the fear as a feeling of anxiety, discomfort, or even relief, depending on how you view the situation.

In summary, emotions are automatic, biological responses to stimuli, while feelings are the conscious interpretations of those emotions. Emotions are universal and short lived, serving as a vital part of our survival mechanisms. Feelings, however, are shaped by personal experiences and can linger long after the initial emotional response. By understanding the difference between the two, you can better navigate your emotional landscape and develop more effective ways to manage your thoughts, reactions, and wellbeing.

Anxiety and PTSD can easily start to feel like they define you, especially when the symptoms are constant and overwhelming. When you're living with daily stress, panic attacks, or flashbacks, it's easy to begin seeing yourself as "an anxious person" or someone who's "trapped" by trauma. Over time, these conditions can become part of your identity, and you might start to believe that this is just who you are. However, it's important to remember that while anxiety and PTSD are part of your experience, THEY DON'T DEFINE YOU.

Here's how anxiety and PTSD can take over your identity:
- **Constant Symptoms**: The regular presence of anxiety or PTSD can make it feel like these conditions dominate every part of your life.
- **Self–Labeling**: You might start seeing yourself as your condition, like thinking, "I am anxious" rather than "I experience anxiety."

- **Reinforcement from Others**: Sometimes, others treat you differently, reinforcing the idea that your condition defines you. Even though it's uncomfortable, living with anxiety or PTSD can feel safer than facing the unknown, making it hard to let go of that identity.

Vicious Cycle of panic

Situation (trigger)
Such as being somewhere crowded like a supermarket or on a bus

Thoughts
- Intense anxiety
- Scared
- Very frightened and in danger

Feel in danger 'flight or fight' response is triggered

Feelings
- Intense anxiety
- Scared
- Very frightened and in danger

Cycle continues

Catastrophic misinterpretation of physical sensations

Chatstrophic misinterpretation of physical sensations
- I feel dizzy so I must be going to faint'
- I'm going to stop breathing'
- I'm losing my mind'

Behaviours

Fear gets worse

Rely on safety behaviours to reduce anxiety such as
- Only go to supermarket late at night
- Carry water bottle and stress remedy around at all times
- Only travel on buses with a friend

Leave or avoid situation
- Leave crowded place when feeling panicky
- Avoid town centre
- Avoid places where had a panic attack before

Again, instead of saying **"I am anxious,"** try saying, **"I experience anxiety."** This small shift helps remind you that anxiety is just part of what you deal with, not who you are.

YOU'RE MUCH MORE THAN YOUR MENTAL HEALTH STRUGGLES.

Focus on your other qualities, your interests and skills, and positive traits that have nothing to do with anxiety or trauma. Be kind to yourself. Understand that you're doing the best you can, and feeling anxiety or trauma doesn't mean you're weak or broken.

Anxiety and PTSD can create negative thoughts like "I'll never get better." Start questioning these beliefs. With therapy and support, you can reframe these thoughts and see a path forward. Therapy is essential for managing anxiety and PTSD. Treatments like CBT or EMDR can help you reprocess trauma and retrain your brain to deal with stress in a healthier way. Surround yourself with people who see you for more than your struggles. Positive relationships can remind you of your worth beyond anxiety or PTSD. Mindfulness and grounding exercises can help you stay in the present moment, preventing you from getting lost in past trauma or future worries.

Something that I haven't used much at all but is a technique that has been used and seems to help people is a grounding technique where you focus on your surroundings. Name 5 things you can see, four things you can feel, three things you can hear, two things you can smell and one thing you can taste. I came across this after moving beyond having panic situations and I no longer need or have had the chance to try it out. It seems like it's a great way to tell your mind and subconscious that there is no lurking danger present and it's safe to feel calm. Try it out and see if it might be helpful for you!

Mental Shift:

Don't think of fear as something you always need to run from—think of it as something you can learn to handle in a healthy way. If you find yourself in fear, stress, or anxiety—whether or not it feels rational—pause and ask yourself: *Do I really need to escape this feeling, or do I simply need to help my body become more capable of handling this level of stress?* Instead of reacting with avoidance, shift the question to: *Why is my body struggling to deal with this amount of stress or anxiety?*

This simple reframing can start to move you toward resilience, rather than fear of the fear itself. I want to remind you that this is directly related to the nutrition section as well. The gut microbiome, nervous system (in other words the gut–brain axis) play a role in how you manage anxiety and PTSD. Remember, anxiety and PTSD are part of your journey, but they don't define you. With the right tools, support, and mindset, you can reclaim your identity and live a full, meaningful life beyond these conditions.

Emotional Tone Scale:

Understanding the emotional tone scale is a powerful tool in self-awareness and emotional regulation, especially when working through trauma, PTSD, or long-standing stress patterns. Emotions exist on a spectrum, and while we're often taught to see feelings like anger or sadness as "bad," this scale shows that each emotion has its place and progression. It's not about suppressing how you feel, it's about recognizing where you are and learning how to move toward healthier, more empowering emotional states.

1. Joy/Appreciation/Empowered/Freedom/Love
2. Passion
3. Enthusiasm/Eagerness/Happiness
4. Positive Expectation/Belief
5. Optimism
6. Hopefulness
7. Contentment
8. Boredom
9. Pessimism
10. Frustration/Irritation/Impatience
11. Overwhelm
12. Disappointment
13. Doubt
14. Worry
15. Blame
16. Discouragement
17. Anger
18. Revenge
19. Hatred/Rage
20. Jealousy
21. Insecurity/Guilt/Unworthiness
22. Fear/Grief/Depression/Despair/Powerlessness

For example, anger is often seen as negative, but on the emotional tone scale, it actually sits *above* fear, apathy, and shame. If someone is chronically in fear or guilt, moving into anger can actually be a step toward healing. Anger carries energy, momentum, and the potential for transformation. It means you're no longer frozen or helpless. The goal isn't to stay stuck in anger, but to see it as a phase in the journey upward toward courage, acceptance, and ultimately peace. By understanding this emotional ladder, we stop judging ourselves for how we feel and instead start climbing—one rung at a time.

Let's bring it all together

I want to remind you up front that I'm not a neurochemistry expert or a psychiatrist. What I am is someone who's spent the last 25 years relentlessly studying and applying these ideas—both in my own recovery and in helping others. The following is a distillation of the research and insights I've found most compelling, and I'm excited to share it with you here.

Now that you've gained a basic grasp of PTSD and how the nervous system functions under stress, let's take a closer look at the underlying pathophysiology and neurochemistry. We'll weave together the many strands—HPA axis dysregulation, chronic sympathetic activation, fear, panic, and anxiety—into a single, cohesive picture. From there, you can see how an overtaxed stress response contributes not only to PTSD but also to long-term health issues: depression, sleep disturbances, a weakened immune system, digestive imbalances, and the muscle-memory of living in perpetual fight-or-flight mode. This spider-web of interconnected systems reveals why treating trauma at its roots is essential for restoring true balance and vitality.

When you encounter a threat—whether it's a real danger or a memory that feels just as vivid—your brain and body kick off a rapid, coordinated neurochemical response designed to keep you alive. In someone with PTSD or panic disorder, this system can become hypersensitive, overreacting to cues that most people would easily shrug off.

Here's a straightforward breakdown of what happens behind the scenes:

1. **Amygdala "Alarm Bell" and Glutamate Surge**

   The amygdala is your brain's threat-detector. The moment it perceives danger, it releases the excitatory neurotransmitter glutamate. Glutamate speeds up communication between neurons, ensuring that your alarm bell sounds immediately. In PTSD, the amygdala often becomes over–responsive, so even mildly stressful situations trigger a full alarm.

2. **HPA Axis Activation: CRH → ACTH → Cortisol**

   Almost instantly, the hypothalamus secretes corticotropin-releasing hormone (CRH), which signals the pituitary gland to release adrenocorticotropic hormone (ACTH). ACTH then travels through your bloodstream to the adrenal glands atop your kidneys, prompting them to pump out cortisol—the body's main stress hormone. Cortisol raises blood sugar, sharpens alertness, and temporarily suppresses non–essential functions like digestion and immune responses. In PTSD, this HPA axis loop can become "stuck" on high, so baseline cortisol levels remain elevated and normal feedback mechanisms (which should shut off CRH release) become blunted.

3. **Sympathetic Surge: Epinephrine & Norepinephrine**

   Concurrently, your adrenal medulla floods the bloodstream with epinephrine (adrenaline) and norepinephrine (noradrenaline). These catecholamines accelerate your heart rate, widen your airways, and boost blood flow to muscles—classic "fight or flight" chemistry. In panic disorder, surges of these chemicals can occur unpredictably, causing sudden bouts of racing heart, sweating, and dizziness.

4. **GABA and Serotonin Imbalance**

   Under normal circumstances, the inhibitory neurotransmitter GABA (gamma–aminobutyric acid) and mood-stabilizer serotonin help dial down arousal and restore calm. In PTSD and chronic panic, both systems are often weakened: less GABA means fewer "brakes" on runaway excitation, and altered serotonin signaling can exacerbate anxiety and mood instability.

5. **Pathophysiological Consequences**

Over time, repeated floods of stress hormones and excitatory neurotransmitters can reshape your brain. The hippocampus, critical for contextualizing memories, tends to shrink in chronic stress, which makes it harder to distinguish past trauma from present reality—fueling flashbacks. The prefrontal cortex, which normally puts the brakes on the amygdala, can become less active, weakening your ability to think clearly under pressure.

6. **Putting It All Together**

In PTSD and panic disorder, this neurochemical orchestra plays at full volume far too often. Your body stays locked in a heightened state of alarm, and simple reminders—crowded rooms, loud noises, even certain smells—can trigger the entire cascade again. Understanding these mechanisms is the first step toward targeted interventions—whether that's learning breathing techniques to boost GABA activity, practicing mindfulness to reengage the prefrontal cortex, or seeking therapies that recalibrate your HPA axis and catecholamine balance. With time and the right tools, you can teach your system to recognize real danger and stand down when the coast is clear.

Now, the last thing before we move on is breaking down the freeze response, which is a little different.

Immediate Neurochemistry of Freeze

When neither fight nor flight is possible, the dorsal branch of the vagus nerve floods the body with parasympathetic signals, effectively overriding any urge to move or escape. At the same time, your brain releases natural opioids—endorphins—to numb pain and distress, acting like an internal anesthetic. In some cases of extreme stress, you may even experience a brief spike in oxytocin, which paradoxically promotes a "social–attachment" type of shutdown rather than connection.

Meanwhile, inhibitory neurotransmitters such as GABA rise alongside parasympathetic acetylcholine, further slowing your heart rate and metabolism. The HPA axis may still trigger cortisol release, but its effects become unpredictable—sometimes surging, sometimes dipping—adding to that heavy, "shut–down" sensation.

Pathophysiological Consequences of Freeze

With parasympathetic overdrive, your heart rate and blood pressure can plummet, leading to lightheadedness, "out–of–body" sensations, and emotional numbness. Over time, chronically high dorsal vagal tone acts like an overloaded brake, weakening your ability to shift back into a normal resting state and leaving you stuck in low–energy, immobilized mode. In the brain, the rational prefrontal cortex goes offline while the amygdala stays hyper alert, creating a split between the sensation of being frozen and the knowledge that you're no longer in danger. On the body's systems, prolonged freeze means poor gut motility and nutrient absorption, as well as immune dysregulation.

Parasympathetic dominance may momentarily bolster certain immune functions, but long–term suppression leads to more harm than good. Structurally, repeated freeze episodes contribute to hippocampal shrinkage (making it harder to tag memories with context) and further weaken prefrontal control, cementing the shutdown pattern even more deeply.

Why It Matters

Recognizing these neurochemical "switches" and their

pathophysiological impact explains why you can't simply "snap out of it." True recovery demands both nervous–system retraining through movement-based exercises like martial arts, yoga, somatic exercises, vagal–tone balancing exercises, and brain and mental focused work, such as Cognitive Behavior Therapy.

I want to take a moment to somewhat define "somatic." In the context of PTSD and trauma, "somatic" refers to the body's role in storing, expressing, and ultimately releasing traumatic stress. Rather than focusing solely on thoughts or emotions, somatic approaches recognize that trauma often becomes encoded in physical sensations—tightness in the chest, gut "knots," trembling, or chronic pain. Somatic therapies invite you to bring mindful awareness to these bodily signals—tracking where you feel tension, noticing how it shifts with your breath, and learning gentle movement or touch techniques to help discharge trapped energy. By tuning into and gently working with the body's own wisdom, somatic work can dissolve the felt sense of threat, restore nervous system balance, and integrate mind and body in the healing of PTSD, anxiety, and chronic stress.

I want to reiterate here that consistent reactivation of the freeze response contributes to extreme fatigue, melancholy and some may have more depression. Something that kept me going through all those years of suffering was that I just knew I had to keep going. There was no other option. That was one thing, *that* spark, which kept me going and kept me alive. There was really no other option, anything else was either worse or similar, so I might as well keep going, keep fighting.

To overcome freeze, you need the opposite action. You need to work on the mind (including some things we already went over and lots of good stuff coming in the CBT section). For times when I had fight or flight, I needed some of the opposite of that—to teach my brain, mind and nervous system to calm down and find more parasympathetic relaxation. There's a place for light activity within a fight–or–flight stress response, which we'll get to later on.

Takeaways from Chapter 5

- Once you have the okay from your doctor, assuming you did this step (which I encourage), start to become aware of the symptoms that you're having and just know that they can generally, within reason, come from panic and/or anxiety.
- If you're having intense symptoms of anxiety or panic, please try EFT with Brad Yates, by searching YouTube for his Video – "EFT for Panic" or other videos that might interest you.
- The good stress and that nervousness you can get before going on stage or before job interviews, etc. can help give you more energy and help you to perform better!
- If the nervousness and anxiety are overwhelming and disturbs your life, then this means you've become dysregulated and need deeper healing from, most likely, PTSD and or panic/anxiety disorder.
- Become a little more mindful of any sensations that may come up in the early onset of a panic situation. With what you've already learned, you may be able to talk yourself down. Be mindful of why you may feel a certain way afterwards also. Just knowing this can help.
- The vagus nerve is of upmost importance in your recovery and healing from any kind of panic disorder, pain, PTSD and depression.
- Remember the differences between emotions and feelings and learn to become more aware of the difference. Emotions are automatic, biological responses to stimuli, while feelings are the conscious interpretations of those emotions. Chapter 7 will go deeper in this with Cognitive Behavior Therapy.
- Your anxiety or PTSD, **DOES NOT** define you.
- Check in with yourself using the emotional tone scale—it's a simple yet powerful tool to get a snapshot of where you're at emotionally. Once you identify your current state, see if you can gently shift one level higher. Even moving from apathy to frustration, or fear to anger, can be progress. The goal isn't to

fake happiness, but to build awareness and move upward toward more empowering states, one step at a time.
- If you're interested, learning a little about the neurochemistry and pathophysiology of PTSD and the stress response can be a powerful mental shift when dealing with and overcoming trauma.

Chapter 6
The Breath

"You don't have to control your thoughts. You just have to stop letting them control you."
— Dan Millman

The breath can play a key role in any panic or anxiety situation. It's often one of the most effective tools available and can provide the "anti–venom," so to speak. That said, when I used to experience intense panic, breathing alone wasn't always my best option. In those moments, my mental state—specifically my ability to use cognitive techniques—was more helpful. For others, taking a deep, grounding breath can make all the difference in the world. It really depends on the individual and the situation.

That said, all of the breathwork and training I've done over the years has absolutely helped me—no matter the intensity of what I was going through.

IMPORTANT NOTE:
It's generally best to breathe through the nose. Nose breathing helps humidify and filter the air, and it allows the body to naturally regulate airflow, especially during sleep. Interestingly, blood pressure tends to shift between sides of the body depending on the nostril in use, and nose breathing also promotes the production of nitric oxide, a molecule that supports circulation and cellular health.

Now, let's talk about something important. Some health and psychology experts disagree on the role of breath during panic attacks.

One camp believes that breathwork isn't worth focusing on in the moment of panic; others insist that it's the most powerful tool you have. I've heard both arguments, and here's my take:

Use whatever works. Period. There's no one–size–fits–all solution here. For someone dealing with PTSD, panic disorder, or chronic anxiety, breathwork alone may not be enough, but that doesn't mean it isn't helpful. I recommend combining it with tools like Cognitive Behavioral Therapy (CBT), yoga, and other supportive practices that address both mind and body.

One person might find that taking just a couple of deep belly breaths is enough to bring them down from a level 5 to a level 4. That's a win. That's progress. Even if it's just a baby step, it's a step in the right direction. Deep breathing can help shift your awareness from the racing mind back into your body.

On the other hand, someone else may spiral into panic so fast that they need something stronger to pull their thoughts back on track—whether it's CBT, a grounding technique, or an effective distraction. Every person has to find what works best for them in those moments.

Please trust me when I say that many of the techniques I'm sharing with you have worked, and will continue to work for thousands of people.

You CAN tap into that badass calm and inner peace.

I shared a bit of my story in the introduction but let me revisit it briefly. I know what it's like to feel like anxiety or panic is happening "to you," as if your body is attacking you. But if you've read this far, you already understand that this isn't the full picture.

I know what it's like to feel as if the air is being pulled from your lungs. For me, hyperventilation was my body's default reaction. I used to carry a paper bag everywhere because I never knew when a panic attack might hit. Sometimes I had multiple attacks a day for weeks on end. At the time, I didn't have a job or a family, which was a blessing, because honestly, I don't know how I could've functioned if I had. Looking back, if I had more responsibilities, I probably would've needed medication just to stabilize. I couldn't sleep. I was nearly housebound. I couldn't go anywhere. I even had panic attacks during sex.

Everything I'm sharing in this book helped pull me out of that spiral. These tools brought me back to life—and more than that, they helped me build a thriving one.

Before we move into specific breathing techniques, let's take a moment to go over some simple anatomy behind breath and why it matters so much in times of stress and healing.

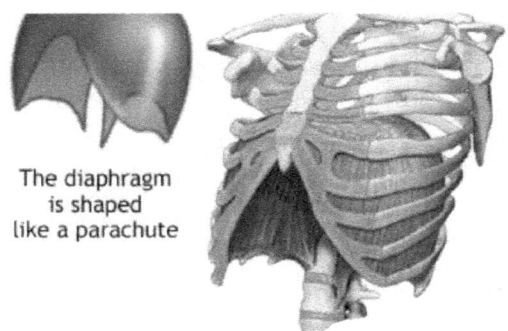

The diaphragm is shaped like a parachute

As you can see in the diagram above, the diaphragm sits tucked up inside the ribcage, just beneath the lungs. When you take in a big sip of air, this dome–shaped muscle contracts and moves downward, creating more space for your lungs to expand. This simple motion is at the core of deep, healthy breathing.

Take a moment now—get comfortable where you're sitting—and try this. Inhale deeply and imagine your diaphragm moving downward toward your lower organs. As you exhale, visualize it rising back up again. Do this a few more times, following the motion with your mind. Just this little awareness can be a calming and powerful breathing technique all by itself.

This is the foundation of what's often called "belly breathing." On the inhale, your diaphragm pushes down, gently pressing on your internal organs, causing your lower belly to expand outward. This creates space for your lungs to fully expand, pulling in more oxygen that is delivered throughout your bloodstream, into your brain, and throughout your entire body.

Most people walk around with stale air trapped in their lungs simply because they're only using a fraction of their total lung capacity. Shallow chest breathing becomes the norm, especially under chronic stress. But deep breathing? That's where healing begins.

Here are just some of the benefits of deep breathing:
- Activates the parasympathetic nervous system, decreasing stress and increasing calm
- Helps to relieve pain
- Stimulates the lymphatic system, supporting the body's natural detox processes
- Strengthens immunity
- Boosts energy levels
- Lowers blood pressure
- Improves digestion
- Supports better posture

Now, if deep breathing feels hard for you, know that you're not alone and that there are valid reasons for this. Many of the challenges come from both physical patterns and nervous system conditioning. Chronic stress is one of the biggest culprits. When we're constantly in fight–or–flight mode (sympathetic dominance), the body defaults to shallow, upper–chest breathing. Over time, this pattern locks the diaphragm in a tight, frozen state, making full breaths feel strained or unnatural.

The muscles around the ribcage can also lose flexibility and strength from disuse. Many people simply aren't used to belly breathing anymore, and even unconsciously resist it, either because it feels too vulnerable or because it's unfamiliar. On top of that, a low vagal tone (poor vagus nerve regulation) can reinforce these shallow breathing patterns, keeping the nervous system stuck in a reactive loop.

The good news? This can be retrained. Restoring your body's natural ability to breathe deeply and calmly just takes a little intention and consistency. By practicing mindful breathing, releasing tension, and reconditioning your nervous system to feel safe in your body, you can begin to reclaim the healing power of your breath. One inhale at a time.

Hyperventilation (You won't be so afraid once you learn this)

It's helpful to understand what is actually happening when someone hyperventilates. Hyperventilation occurs when you breathe more rapidly or deeply than necessary, which can be triggered by stress, anxiety, or panic, among other causes. This excessive breathing leads to several physiological changes in the body, such as:

- **Decrease in carbon dioxide levels**: hyperventilation causes you to exhale more carbon dioxide (CO_2) than your body can produce. This leads to a significant decrease in the level of CO_2 in the blood, a condition known as hypocapnia.

- **Respiratory alkalosis**: with reduced CO_2 levels, the pH of the blood increases, making it more alkaline. This condition is known as respiratory alkalosis. The human body requires a very narrow range of pH to function optimally, and even slight changes can have significant effects (this is why breathing in a bag helps to keep more CO_2 in the blood, because you're breathing back in your own CO_2).

- **Constriction of blood vessels**: lowered CO_2 levels cause the blood vessels to constrict, particularly those supplying blood to the brain. This can lead to symptoms such as lightheadedness, dizziness, rapid heart rate and sometimes fainting.

- **Reduced blood flow to the brain**: constricted blood vessels mean less blood flow to the brain, which can cause cognitive and perceptual disturbances, such as confusion, blurred vision, or a feeling of unreality.

- **Altered calcium and potassium levels**: hyperventilation affects the balance of certain minerals in the blood, particularly calcium and potassium, which can lead to neurological symptoms like tingling in the fingers and around the mouth, muscle cramps, and weakness.

- **Increase in heart rate**: the body may respond to hyperventilation by increasing the heart rate, which can be perceived as heart palpitations or chest pain, further exacerbating feelings of anxiety or panic.

- **Physical symptoms**: other physical symptoms may include sweating, dry mouth, inability to concentrate, and sometimes feelings of suffocation or over–breathing. You might start to swallow a lot due to the anxiety and dried mouth and throat as well.

It's important to note that while hyperventilation is often associated with anxiety or panic attacks, it can also be caused by medical conditions such as asthma, chronic obstructive pulmonary disease (COPD), or heart conditions. Therefore, persistent or recurrent hyperventilation should be evaluated by a healthcare professional.

Practicing Breathwork

Generally, it's best to practice breathwork and deep breathing while sitting or lying down with your knees up. This will give your body and diaphragm an easier time to allow for deeper breathing. Keep in mind you may not want to use any deep breathing techniques if your diaphragm is frozen, or not very flexible, like we spoke about earlier and breathing is difficult. Breathing techniques, especially without proper guidance, can cause lightheadedness and dizziness, amongst other symptoms. Nothing too drastic, but enough to not want to add to your stress and panic symptoms you already might be having.

Try this: if you're having trouble taking deeper breaths or just feel extra tightness in your breathing, try this simple QiGong Breathing Technique. Place your hands on your lower ribs under your chest. As you expand your diaphragm, your lower ribs should expand out. Practice this expansion of the ribs a handful of times, up to a few times a day.

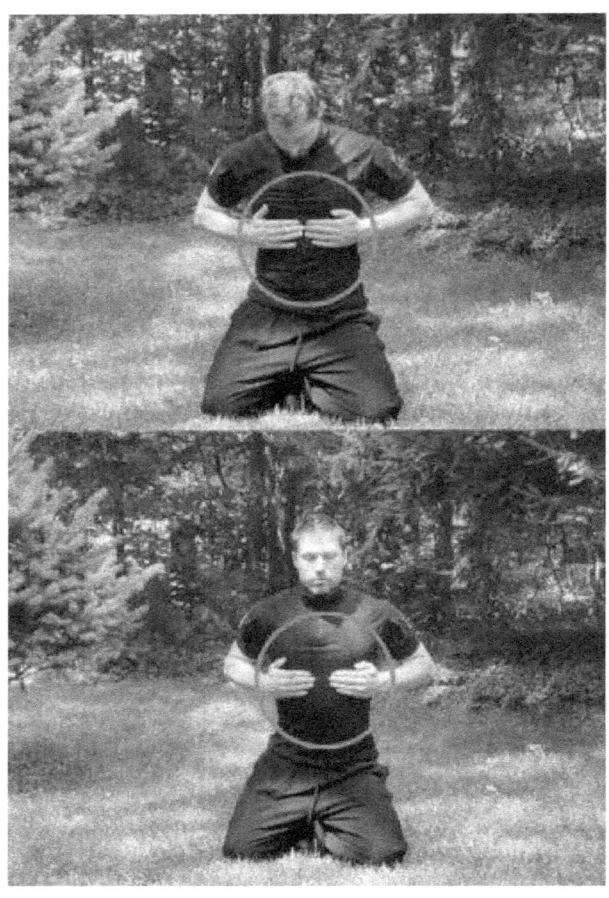

Next try this:

The next technique is very simple and for beginners, but it can be useful to anyone at any time. This is another one I learned from QiGong and still use today. Start by standing comfortably. Roll your shoulders forward slightly, gently bow your head and round the back a little bit.

Start with arms and chest bowed forward and, on the inhale, simply open and expand the chest, open the arms, arch the back, and lift the head. It's very easy, but it can be done anywhere. This technique can feel subtle at first, but the more often you do this, it can feel profound.

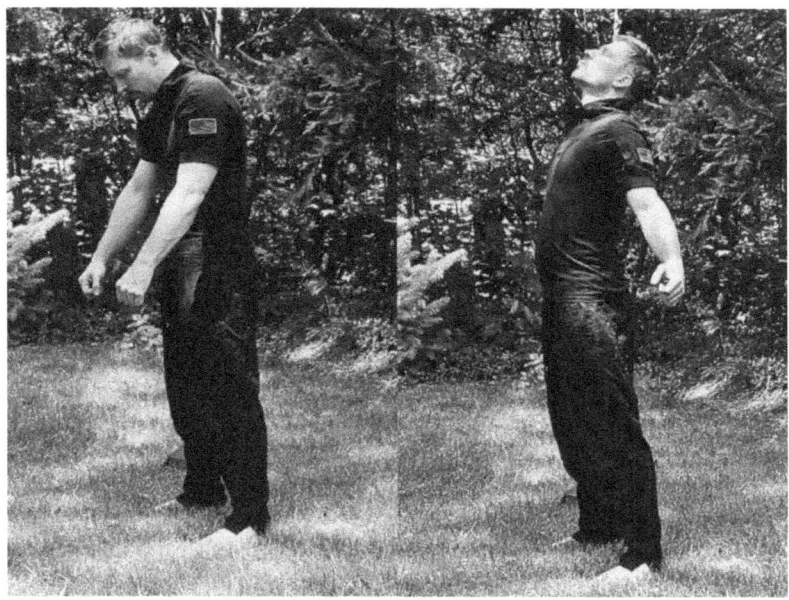

And now this one:

The last technique is also from QiGong. Start on all fours. Place a hand over the belly button. Exhale and tuck the belly up and in and lightly assist with your hand. Now exhale and allow the full drop and relaxation of the diaphragm and allow the lower belly to drop down. Allow yourself to be girthy and round! This might not be easy at first. This helps to release your diaphragm, especially for what's called a "frozen diaphragm" muscle and allow more breath to the lower lungs. This also helps tonify and strengthen the lung and breathing muscles.

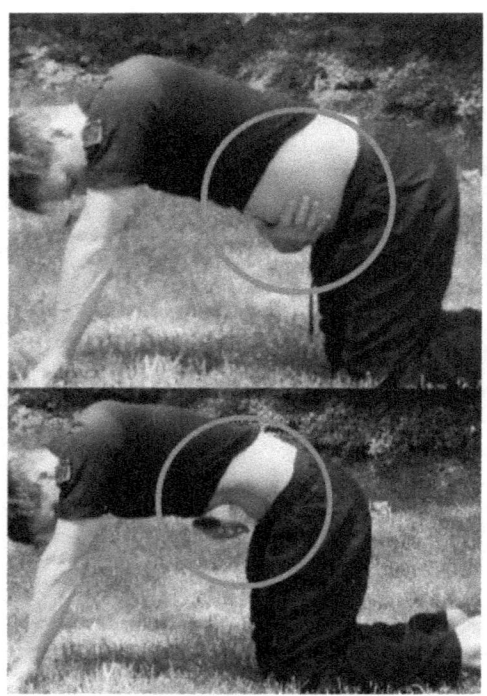

Ujjayi Breath

Let's chat about an ancient breathing method called Ujjayi, which means victorious, powerful. Ujjayi breathing, also known as "victorious breath" or "ocean breath," is a pranayama (breath control) technique commonly practiced in yoga. This breathing method helps to calm the mind, improve concentration, balance the hemispheres of the brain and regulate the flow of prana (life force) in the body. It's really worth watching a how-to video on this, but I will try to explain it here for you.

Steps to Practice Ujjayi Breathing:
1. Sit in a comfortable, upright position. You can sit cross legged on the floor or on a chair with your feet flat on the ground.
2. Relax and settle in. Close your eyes and take a few moments to relax your body.
3. Bring your attention to your breath and allow it to flow naturally.
4. Begin by inhaling deeply through your nose. As you inhale, slightly constrict the back of your throat (glottis). This constriction should create a soft, whispering sound similar to the sound of the ocean.
5. Exhale through your nose while maintaining the slight constriction at the back of your throat. Again, the exhale should produce a soft, oceanic sound. Ensure the breath is smooth and controlled. Imagine that you are fogging up a mirror with your breath, but with your mouth closed.

Create a Rhythm:

Continue breathing in this manner, creating a steady and rhythmic pattern. Aim to make the length of your inhalations and exhalations equal at first. Focus on the sound and sensation of your breath. As this gets easier, start to exhale for longer than the inhale. Inhale for 4 seconds and exhale for 5-6 seconds. Then try to inhale for 4 seconds and exhale for 8 seconds. Performing a longer exhale is a signal to the parasympathetic nervous system to turn on, which will cause you to feel calmer and more relaxed. This also has a vacuum type of signal with your heart. An analog signal versus an electrical signal if you will. This is why and how working with the breath can be so helpful.

Maintain Awareness:

Keep your awareness on your breath, the sound it creates, and the sensations in your body. This mindfulness helps deepen the practice and enhances its calming effects. Some people, depending on the state of the situation, may need to focus more on the mind or something physical to help support their breath practice. Everyone's different.

Tips for Ujjayi Breathing:
- Practice Ujjayi breathing regularly to develop a deeper sense of relaxation and control.
- Try for a minute when you first start. After feeling comfortable, just a few minutes of Ujjayi breathing can bring the body and mind to a place of calm and relaxation.
- The constriction at the back of the throat should be gentle. If you feel any strain, ease off slightly.
- Ujjayi breathing is often used during yoga asana practice to maintain a steady flow of breath and to link breath with movement.

Benefits of Ujjayi Breathing:
- Calms the mind: the rhythmic nature of Ujjayi breathing helps to calm the nervous system and reduce stress.
- Enhances concentration: focusing on the breath increases mindfulness and concentration.
- Regulates prana: It helps regulate the flow of prana (life force) throughout the body.
- Improves oxygenation: deep, controlled breathing improves oxygenation of the blood and enhances overall respiratory efficiency.

By practicing Ujjayi breathing, you can achieve a state of mental clarity, emotional balance, and physical relaxation, enhancing your overall well–being.

Cascade Breathing (Full-Body Expansion)

This technique involves a three-stage inhale and a reverse three-stage exhale. Begin by inhaling into your belly, feeling it expand outward. Next, draw that breath up into your solar plexus (mid-chest), then complete the inhale by filling your upper chest. On the exhale, reverse the pattern: first soften and release your chest, then let your mid-chest collapse back in, and finally pull your belly gently toward your spine. This "cascade" of expansion and contraction helps move breath through the full capacity of your lungs and can be especially powerful for grounding and centering during the day.

Solar-Plexus to Chest Breathing (Daytime Balance)

For a slightly lighter practice, focus your inhale on the area just below your sternum (solar plexus), then lift the breath into your upper chest. When you exhale, let the breath flow back down through the chest and out via the solar plexus. This pattern gives you a deep, energizing breath without fully engaging the parasympathetic "rest-and-digest" response—perfect for mornings or times when you need clarity and alertness.

When to Use Which Breath

Reserve full "belly balloon" breathing (deep diaphragmatic inhale and exhale) for bedtime, pre-meal calm, or whenever you need extra vagal-nerve stimulation. If you find yourself overusing it—especially under chronic stress—you can teeter into excessive parasympathetic activation (feeling overly lethargic or "stuck"). The lighter solar-plexus–to–chest pattern is your go-to for daytime practice, giving you depth without the risk of dysregulating your system.

Takeaways from Chapter 6

- Breath (prana) is our vital life force.
- You don't need to spend endless minutes on pranayama to feel its benefits; often just one or two deep, intentional breaths can shift your state profoundly. That said, if you enjoy a longer practice—one or two minutes of mindful breathing—by all means, lean into it.
- Deep breathing supports your mind, body, and subtle energy in countless ways: it calms stress, enhances focus, and encourages better circulation and digestion.
- In the morning, try a simple three-stage breath—expanding belly, rib cage, then chest—to awaken your system. At meals or before bed, switch to deep belly-balloon breathing to promote relaxation and support healthy vagal tone.
- Understanding how your diaphragm works—how it contracts downward on the inhale and relaxes upward on the exhale—will help you breathe more fully and reap the full rewards of each breath.

Chapter 7
Cognitive Behavior Therapy

"The greatest sources of our suffering are the lies we tell ourselves."
— *Bessel A. van der Kolk*

Cognitive Behavioral Therapy (CBT) is a form of psychological treatment that has been demonstrated to be effective for a range of problems including PTSD, C-PTSD, depression, anxiety disorders, alcohol and drug use problems, marital problems, eating disorders, severe mental illness, phobias and more.

Psychiatrist Dr. Aaron T. Beck developed CBT in the 1960s based on the idea that our thoughts, feelings, and behaviors are deeply interconnected. He discovered that people with depression and anxiety often experience distorted, automatic negative thoughts that shape their emotional responses and behavior. The goal is to help individuals become more aware of their inner dialogue, shift their mindset, and break the cycle of emotional suffering. CBT is practical, goal–oriented and backed by decades of clinical research.

CBT focuses on identifying and challenging those unhelpful thought patterns, called cognitive distortions, and replacing them with more realistic, empowering beliefs. Through structured exercises, clients learn to:
- Recognize distorted thinking (like catastrophizing or black–and–white, extreme thinking)
- Evaluate those thoughts objectively
- Develop healthier responses and behaviors
- Understand what might be causing anxiety and where PTSD may be coming from

We will be covering many areas of CBT in this section. There are volumes and volumes of information on CBT, so if you take a liking to it, there is a lot out there for you. Here, we will dive just a bit into CBT, but it's enough for you to get started.

Cognitive Distortions

Cognitive distortions are internal mental filters or biases that increase our misery, fuel our anxiety, and make us feel bad about ourselves. Why do we have them? We have them because they have been trained into us from birth. They become our belief systems. We "learn" them from parents, friends, siblings, teachers, social media and more. They are mental patterns of thinking that become what we believe and perceive about ourselves, others and our environment. They are also tied closely to our cognitive biases, which we will cover next. **While reading through these, think how they might apply to you in your life.**

IMPORTANT NOTE:
Our first seven years are critically important, as this is when our nervous system undergoes its most significant development. The experiences we have during this period set the foundation for the rest of our lives. Understanding this, especially for parents, is essential for nurturing healthy, resilient children.

The following is a list of common cognitive distortions and their definitions:

Filtering: Mental filtering is when your mind fixates on the negative aspects of a situation while filtering out or ignoring anything positive. Even if there are more good things than bad, your attention zeroes in on what's wrong, creating a distorted and overly negative perception

Polarization: Polarized thinking is thinking about yourself and the world in an "all–or–nothing" way. When you engage in thoughts in black or white, with no shades of gray, this type of cognitive distortion is leading you. All or nothing thinking usually leads to extremely unrealistic standards for yourself and others that could affect your relationships and motivation. Black–or–white thoughts may also set you up for failure. When you engage in polarized thinking, everything is in "either/or" categories. This might make you miss the complexity of most people and situations.

Overgeneralization: When you overgeneralize something, you take an isolated negative event and turn it into a never–ending pattern of loss and defeat. With overgeneralization, words like "always," "never," "everything," and "nothing" are frequent in your train of thought. Overgeneralization can also manifest in your thoughts about the world and its events.

Discounting the positive: Discounting positives is closely related to mental filtering, but with a key distinction: instead of simply overlooking the positive, you acknowledge it—then immediately dismiss it as meaningless or undeserved. For example, if someone compliments your work, you might think, "they're just being nice," or "anyone could've done it." This habit of downplaying or rejecting positive feedback or achievements prevents you from fully internalizing success or building self–confidence. Over time, it reinforces a mindset that nothing you do is ever truly good enough.

Jumping to conclusions: When you jump to conclusions, you interpret an event or situation negatively without evidence supporting such a conclusion. Then you react to your assumption, not what has happened. Jumping to conclusions or "mindreading" is often in response to a persistent thought or concern of your own.

Catastrophizing: Catastrophizing is related to jumping to conclusions. In this case, you jump to the worst possible conclusion in every scenario, no matter how improbable it is. This cognitive distortion often comes with "what if" questions. What if he didn't call because he got into an accident? What if she hadn't arrived because she really didn't want to spend time with me? What if I help this person and they end up betraying or abandoning me? Several questions might arise in response to one event.

Personalization: Personalization leads you to believe that you're responsible for events that, in reality, are completely or partially out of your control. This cognitive distortion often results in you feeling guilty or assigning blame without contemplating all factors involved. With personalizing, you also take things personally when they aren't personal.

Control fallacies: The word fallacy refers to an illusion, misconception, or error. Control fallacies can go two opposite ways: you either feel responsible or in control of everything in your life, or you feel you have no control over anything in your life. The other type of control fallacy is based on the belief that your actions and presence impact or control the lives of others.

Fallacy of fairness: This cognitive distortion refers to measuring every behavior and situation on a scale of fairness. Finding that other people don't assign the same value of fairness to the event makes you resentful. In other words, you believe you know what's fair and what isn't, and it upsets you when other people disagree with you. The fallacy of fairness will lead you to face conflict with certain people and situations because you feel the need for everything to be "fair" according to your own parameters. But fairness is rarely absolute and can often be self-serving.

Blaming: Blaming refers to making others responsible for how you feel. "You made me feel bad" is what usually defines this cognitive distortion. However, even when others engage in hurtful behaviors, you're still in control of how you feel in most situations. The distortion comes from believing that others have the power to affect your life, even more than you.

Shoulds: As cognitive distortions, "should" statements are subjective ironclad rules you set for yourself and others without considering the specifics of a circumstance. You tell yourself that things should be a certain way with no exceptions. When it comes to yourself, you might believe you should always make your bed, or you should always make people laugh. "You should be better," you constantly tell yourself. When these things don't happen—they really depend on many factors— you feel guilty, disappointed, let down, or frustrated. You may believe you're trying to motivate yourself with these statements, such as "I should go to the gym every day." However, when circumstances change, and you can't do what you "should," you become angry and upset. You got out of work late and couldn't get to the gym, for example.

Emotional Reasoning: Emotional reasoning leads you to believe that the way you feel reflects reality. "I feel this way about this situation; therefore, it must be a fact," defines this cognitive distortion. This cognitive distortion might also lead you to believe future events depend on how you feel. You might also assess a random situation based on your emotional reaction. If someone says something that makes you angry, you immediately conclude that person is treating you poorly.

Fallacy of change: The fallacy of change involves believing that other people will adjust their behavior to meet your expectations, especially if you push or pressure them hard enough. This mindset assumes that your happiness or peace depends on someone else changing, rather than accepting them as they are or setting healthy boundaries. It often leads to frustration, resentment, and strained relationships, as the focus stays on controlling others instead of managing your own reactions and choices.

Global labeling: Labeling or mislabeling refers to taking a single attribute and turning it into an absolute. This happens when you judge and then define yourself or others based on an isolated event. The labels assigned are usually negative and extreme. This is an extreme form of overgeneralization that leads you to judge an action without taking the context into account. This, in turn, leads you to see yourself and others in ways that might not be accurate. Assigning labels to others can impact how you interact with them. This, in turn, could add friction to your relationships. When you assign those labels to yourself, it can hurt your self-esteem and confidence, leading you to feel insecure and anxious.

Always being right: This desire turns into a cognitive distortion when it trumps everything else, including evidence and other people's feelings. In this cognitive distortion, you see your own opinions as facts of life. This is why you will go to great lengths to prove you're right.

Automatic thoughts: Automatic thoughts are quick, involuntary, and often not fully articulated in the mind and arise in response to specific stimuli or situations. They can be positive, neutral, or negative. In the context of PTSD and anxiety, automatic thoughts are predominantly negative and can significantly impact a person's mental health and wellbeing.

Automatic thoughts are a natural part of the cognitive process and can shape our emotional and behavioral responses. In individuals with PTSD and anxiety, these thoughts are usually distorted and irrational, contributing to the persistence and exacerbation of symptoms. For individuals with PTSD, automatic thoughts often stem from traumatic experiences. These thoughts can include vivid memories of the trauma, self-blame, and negative beliefs about oneself and the world. The thoughts are typically intrusive and can be triggered by reminders of the traumatic event, leading to flashbacks, nightmares, and heightened anxiety.

Andrew Bustamante (ex-CIA Intel officer) talks about how when something happens outside of us or in response to a stimulus, automatic thoughts happen in our mind. When this happens, both sides of our brain take these thoughts in at the same time and try to interpret it. The emotional brain is quicker to interpret it because of our ancestral stress response in fight or flight or freeze. Understanding that our brains do this is where we can get into some real transformation. We can learn how to slow down our emotional brain response and we can work to have our logical brain respond with more control. The techniques in this book will help you learn how to calm the emotional brain and speed up and logical brain so that you can start the process of stopping the anxiety loop from happening or from getting out of control.

Examples of Automatic Thoughts in PTSD
- Re-experiencing the trauma: "I'm back in that terrible situation."
- Self-blame: "It was my fault; I should have done something differently."
- Negative Worldview: "The world is a dangerous place; I can never be safe."

These thoughts perpetuate the cycle of distress, making it difficult for individuals to move past the traumatic event and leading to chronic anxiety and hyperarousal.

Automatic Thoughts in Anxiety – Its Nature and Impact

In anxiety disorders, automatic thoughts are often related to fear and anticipation of future threats. These thoughts can lead to excessive worry and physical symptoms of anxiety, such as increased heart rate and sweating. They're typically characterized by catastrophizing, overgeneralization, and black-and-white thinking.

Examples of Automatic Thoughts in Anxiety
- Catastrophizing: "If I fail this exam, my life will be ruined."
- Overgeneralization: "I made a mistake at work; I'm terrible at my job."
- Black-and-White Thinking: "If I'm not perfect, I'm a complete failure."

Such thoughts can lead to avoidance behaviors, further entrenching anxiety and preventing individuals from engaging in everyday activities.

CBT is a widely used therapy for addressing automatic thoughts in PTSD and anxiety. The process involves:

- Identification: helping individuals become aware of their automatic thoughts.
- Evaluation: assessing the validity of these thoughts and their impact on emotions and behaviors.
- Modification: challenging and restructuring these thoughts to be more balanced and realistic.

Techniques Used in CBT
1. Cognitive Restructuring: identifying and challenging distorted thoughts, replacing them with more accurate and constructive ones.
2. Thought Records: keeping a journal of automatic thoughts, emotions, and alternative responses.
3. Behavioral Experiments: testing the validity of negative thoughts through real–life experiments and observations.

Automatic thoughts play a significant role in the maintenance of PTSD and anxiety disorders. By understanding and addressing these thoughts through therapeutic interventions like CBT, individuals can learn to manage their symptoms more effectively and improve their overall mental health.

I know you can do at least some of this work on your own but understand that it's very helpful to work with a professional as well. The process of identifying, evaluating, and modifying automatic thoughts is crucial for breaking the cycle of negative thinking and fostering resilience and recovery.

So, what you can start doing (and this can be difficult) is when an automatic thought comes up, immediately write it down. Maybe make a special folder on your phone or carry a small notebook with you. That's the first step. Just becoming aware of the thoughts is a huge step. This was difficult for me at first. It will be very helpful if you have this list when you go into therapy or talk with someone you trust to support and help you. Even Andrew Bustamante talks about how important and powerful it is, because it engages your nervous system and engages both sides of your brain at the same time.

Socratic questioning

> **PANIC TO POTENTIAL TOOL**
> You'll want to save this spot so you can reference it later when you're doing journal entries. Journal templates can be found at the end of this chapter.

Socratic questioning is a disciplined method of questioning that is deeply rooted in the teaching techniques of Socrates, an ancient Greek philosopher. It involves asking a series of questions not only to draw out individual answers but also to encourage fundamental insight into the issues at hand. This method is widely used in various fields such as psychology, education, psychotherapy, law, and everyday life to foster critical thinking, uncover underlying assumptions, explore and interpret ideas, analyze concepts, distinguish what we know from what we don't, and help us follow the logical implications of how we think. It's a great way to pursue our thoughts in many directions and for many purposes.

Key Characteristics:
1. Systematic: following a structured approach, aiming to delve deeper into the subject matter.
2. Focused: targeted and specific questioning, often honing in on one aspect of the topic.
3. Open-ended: questions that are designed to be thought-provoking rather than getting simple yes/no answers.
4. Exploratory: explore underlying beliefs, assumptions, and evidence.

Socratic questions for automatic thinking:

Try not to get overwhelmed by the list of questions. This process can be tough, but honestly, it's where some really good solid therapy happens. With that said, pick just one question or a few—ones that resonate or jump out for you and start there. You can always come back to this list.

1. What evidence do I have that this thought is true? AND is it ABSOLUTELY TRUE?
2. What evidence do I have that this thought is not true?
3. What would a friend say about this thought?
4. What is the worst that could happen? How would I cope if it did?
5. Am I confusing a thought with a fact? Am I confusing an emotion with a fact?
6. How likely is it that my fear will come true?
7. What is the most realistic outcome?
8. Is this thought helpful? Does it serve me?
9. What is the best outcome that could happen?
10. What might be a more balanced way to think about this situation?
11. Am I overestimating the danger or the likelihood of something bad happening?
12. Am I underestimating my ability to cope?
13. Have I been in a similar situation before? How did it turn out?
14. What would I say to someone else who had this thought?
15. What would a trusted mentor or advisor say about this thought?
16. Is there another way of looking at this situation?
17. Am I looking at the whole picture?
18. What are the advantages and disadvantages of thinking this way?
19. Am I blaming myself for something that isn't my fault?
20. Am I taking responsibility for something that is outside my control?

These questions can help to identify, challenge, and reframe negative automatic thoughts, leading to more balanced and rational thinking patterns. So, once you have identified an automatic thought and written it in your journal, you can start the questioning and answering process. You don't have to answer every question so just do your best and it will get easier the more you do it. After a while you might, like me, be able to just have a short conversation within yourself and overcome some or all of the anxiety that came up with the automatic thoughts. In a weird way it can actually be kind of interesting to learn about yourself in this way.

For example, you can start your journal entry like this:
July 10, 2024 – 2:00 p.m., I'm lying in bed (you can state how you're feeling, anxious, guilty etc. and how intense the emotion is. I've used a 1–10 scale, 10 being the most extreme feeling of the emotion)

Thought(s):
I have to get my paper done for Monday and if I don't do a perfect job, I'm going to get fired, no one will like me, I will feel guilty, people depend on me, doom scenario will happen, spiraling, no one will love me, I shame myself and so on and so forth...

Ok, let's break this down, one thought or belief at a time (you can even start writing out thoughts like I'm doing right here). What will actually happen if I don't finish the paper? Now if this is an actual deadline for work or school, then you probably should finish your work and be ready for Monday, BUT does it need to be PERFECT? Probably not. OR how can you get help to make it better? Do you have trouble asking for help from others?

Just start going down more of the Socratic questions and see which ones apply to each situation. This starts to bring you out of your emotional brain and into your logical brain.

Let's say you just do a mediocre job, but it ended up sufficing. All that doom and gloom, guilt, shame, and anxiety happened because you believed somewhere in yourself that if you don't do a perfect job then this cascade of judgment and catastrophizing is going to play out. I just randomly made this story up, but this is how powerful journaling can be. By organizing your thoughts and getting your mind right will help you to make better and more efficient decisions.

For the automatic thoughts and Socratic questioning, you can journal however it works for you, sometimes it could be a page long or more! Sometimes it's just some quick thoughts and maybe a question or two. You don't have to answer everything in the moment, just jotting things down and coming back to it later can be very helpful!

The 5 Questioning *strategy* for PTSD, anxiety and or panic disorders and generalized therapy

This is an alternate Socratic questioning method used by Dr. Daniel Amen, a psychiatrist and brain disorder specialist, that may be helpful. Take whatever is bothering you through this process:

1. Is it true?
2. Is it absolutely true?
3. Three parts: how does the thought make me feel? How does the thought make me act? What's the outcome in believing it's always going to be bad?
4. How would you feel/ act if you didn't have the thought? And the outcome of not having the thought?
5. Take the thought and turn it into the opposite and ask is that true?

The Socratic type questioning method can be tough. It's not easy for people to do this. Take it one step at a time and don't be too hard on yourself, give yourself grace. BUT people do this, and it helps. I did this and still do—it's an ongoing practice and it gets easier. I do it much, much less than I used to for sure, but it's a great tool. Once you can get through the first struggles with your emotions and understanding that you CAN think one way or another and you CAN change your beliefs and mindset, you can see true transformation to your mindset. You can then start to alter your negative beliefs and belief systems.

Start small and before you know it, you'll have a whole journal page of organized thoughts, questioning things that keep you in a limited, narrow mindset that keeps you from being even more successful. Organizing your thoughts is one of the best tools. It puts you in your left brain and helps you to get out of your spiraling emotions.

Cognitive Diffusion

This is about looking AT your thoughts, rather than FROM them. Noticing them rather than getting caught up or buying into them. Letting thoughts come and go rather than holding onto them. This ties into what I spoke about earlier about how our brains work in regard to anxiety and stress. How our brain interprets information and slows down the emotional brain and activating the logical brain first. This partly applies to the Socratic questioning. A quick example would be, "wow I really just had that thought? Thats weird, I don't want to think like that!"

A–B–C–D–E of Cognitive Behavioral Therapy

A: Activating Event (something happens to or around someone)
B: Belief (the event causes someone to have a belief, either rational or irrational)
C: Consequence (the belief leads to a consequence, with rational beliefs leading to healthy consequences and irrational beliefs leading to unhealthy consequences)
D: Disputation (if one has held an irrational belief that has caused unhealthy consequences, they must dispute that belief and turn it into a rational belief)
E: New Effect (the disputation has turned the irrational belief into a rational belief, and the person now has healthier consequences of their belief as a result)

Let's start with A, the activating event. Someone cuts you off in traffic. For conversation's sake, they don't do it on purpose, it was an accident. But this triggers you, you become angry and upset, and for some, maybe even anxious.

Now, most people jump from A to C, skipping the B. C is the consequence, the emotional outburst you may have (anger, anxiety, etc.), basically going straight from the triggering event straight to the emotions. It's no mystery why this happens, we all do it (some more than others) and we often see others do it. After working on this for years, I can now keep a level head in pretty much any situation because I've practiced it so much.

Since you now know how the brain works, you know that the B is where the logical brain comes in. B is the belief and exploring the underlying belief you may have. Since you had an irrational emotional response to the triggering event, then most likely you have an irrational cognitive belief or thinking pattern that led to the irrational (or in some cases, a disproportionate) response. For example, "that jerk swerved in front of me!" So, to work on the B, you might take a moment to THINK about the belief and automatic thoughts, which often go together. You might think (irrationally), people are always swerving around me or "after me" out on the road. Again, our brains can come up the darnedest of things! Or maybe you wonder, "do people even see me!?!" The list goes on. So, what we do is practice with our journals and past situations so that when these moments arise, we can be cool, calm, and collected and use our thinking brains instead of our emotional brains too much.

Instead, what if we were to think, "oh they must be new around here and almost missed the exit and had to get in front of me to get over" (now maybe it's best for them to take the next exit instead of putting others in danger, but we can still influence our automatic thoughts this way, since there wasn't an accident and we can't change the past anyway). Another example, "what if they were a little older and their reaction time is slower?" "What if in their minds there was plenty of room to get over," and you just like to have more space to feel comfortable. The response is totally understandable, but we all live together, we can't all have it our own way.)

"D" is the disputing the irrational thoughts and beliefs. The examples above show how you can dispute the irrational thoughts and beliefs. You could do the same thing with your anxious thoughts and panic feelings.

"E" stands for effect, which is the outcome of disputing irrational thoughts and beliefs. By replacing these irrational thoughts with rational ones, you can respond differently to the triggering event. This helps prevent the roller coaster of emotions and anxiety typically experienced.

Example Scenario: A student receives a low grade on an exam.
1. Activating Event: low grade on the exam.
2. Belief: "I'm a failure and will never succeed."
3. Consequence: feeling depressed and considering dropping out.
4. Disputation: "Is this one grade a true reflection of my abilities? Have I done well in other exams?"
5. Effect: realizing that one school grade doesn't define overall ability, "I'm feeling motivated to study harder."

Conclusion:

The ABCDE Model helps break down complex emotional responses into manageable parts. By understanding and challenging irrational thoughts, you can develop more balanced and rational ways of thinking, leading to better emotional and behavioral outcomes.

Example scenario: A person experiences a panic attack while shopping in a crowded mall.
- **A**ctivating Event: the person is in a crowded mall and starts to feel overwhelmed by the noise and the number of people.
- **B**elief: the person starts thinking, "I can't breathe. I'm going to pass out. I'm losing control. Everyone is staring at me." "I don't feel safe for so and so reasons." "Everyone's judging and looking at me." (This kind of stuff takes work and time and figure out root causes and fix the underlying issue.)
- Emotional **C**onsequences: the person feels intense fear and anxiety. Behavioral **C**onsequences: The person quickly leaves the mall, avoids crowded places in the future, and experiences increased anxiety about having another panic attack.
- **D**isputation: The therapist helps the person challenge, dispute

and question these irrational beliefs by reflecting on whether these are rational thoughts and beliefs.
- **Evidence:** "What evidence do you have that you will pass out or lose control?" "What evidence do you have that *everyone* was staring at you or judging you?"

Alternative Explanations:
- Could it be that your body is reacting to stress rather than a real, immediate danger?
- Is it possible that this is PTSD at play—a familiar trigger causing your body to repeat a stress response it has learned over time, even though the current situation isn't actually threatening?

Rational Response: "Just because I *feel* like I can't breathe doesn't mean I *will* pass out. I've felt this way before, and every time, I've come through it safely. My body is reacting, not failing."

Effect: The person's response to the triggering event changes. They begin to think more rationally about the situation.

New Belief: "I'm feeling anxious because I'm overwhelmed, but I can manage this. I've been through it before and was fine."

New Consequences:
- Emotional: reduced fear and anxiety.
- Behavioral: the person might take deep breaths, remind themselves of the rational responses, and continue shopping without leaving the mall.

Step–by–Step Application:
- **Identify the Activating Event**: notice that the panic attack started in the crowded mall.
- **Explore the Belief**: recognize the automatic thoughts ("I'm going to pass out"). It really helps if you have help from someone qualified or a loved one, for help through this.
- **Observe the Consequences**: notice the emotional and behavioral responses (fear, leaving the mall).

- **Engage in Disputation**: challenge the irrational beliefs with questions and alternative explanations.
- **Evaluate the Evidence**: think about what evidence you have that you will experience something negative like passing out. Feel the change in emotion and behavior as the irrational thoughts are replaced with rational ones.

In conclusion, using the ABCDE model helps individuals with panic and anxiety understand the connection between their thoughts and feelings and learn to challenge and change irrational beliefs. This leads to more rational thinking and healthier emotional and behavioral responses, reducing the frequency and intensity of panic attacks.

Anytime a scenario comes up, triggering automatic thoughts come up, and anxiety and negative sensations come up, try to write them down and journal. Then be curious, be interested in the thoughts and sensations. You might find yourself thinking, "wow I just had those thoughts?"

DON'T WORRY, most of us have weird crazy doom and gloom thoughts. We're not all monks with years of heavy meditation to keep the mind calm all the time. Here's a little secret. They might not even be your thoughts. The thoughts might have come through parents, teachers, friends, or social media. Sometimes we don't know why we have certain thoughts, so it's definitely worth exploring.

When we are young, we are very impressionable. We believe what we are told and what beliefs, morals, values that are instilled in us. Sometimes that is just where we get the inner beliefs that a lot of times do us a disservice. We have to uncover them, explore them and get rid of or change them so they are not taking us for a wild goose chase. You know what this is called? "Changing your mind" about something. You literally just think about the certain belief and you can just conversate and or journal, "why do I think that? I don't think that's true, and I'm changing my mind about that right now."

NOTE: We'll revisit this topic and explore how to apply it in everyday life in more detail in Chapter 11.

Cognitive Biases

The last Psychology and Cognitive Behavioral topic is Cognitive Biases. **This is, in my opinion, one of the most important topics in psychology.** Let's chat about it.

Cognitive biases are mental shortcuts our brains use to process information quickly, but they can sometimes lead to errors in judgment. When you read through these, try and take a moment and see where you might have done this or are doing this, in your life. That's how change and reflection is done. That's how you increase self-awareness and awareness of others and environments. And THAT'S how you heal.

Confirmation bias happens when people seek out information that supports what they already believe while ignoring or dismissing anything that contradicts it. This can make it harder to change opinions, even when presented with new evidence. For example, if someone believes a certain diet is the best, they may only read articles that support their view and disregard studies that suggest otherwise. Overcoming confirmation bias requires actively considering different perspectives and being open to changing one's mind when presented with strong evidence.

Availability bias occurs when people judge how likely or important something is based on how easily they can recall examples. If a person frequently hears about shark attacks in the news, they might assume they are common, even though the actual risk is very low. This bias can lead to unnecessary fears or poor decision-making because our memories do not always reflect reality. To counter this, it helps to look at actual statistics and broader patterns instead of relying on personal experiences or sensationalized stories.

Anchoring bias happens when people rely too much on the first piece of information they receive when making a decision. For example, if a store lists a jacket at $200 but then offers a sale price of $100, people may think they're getting a great deal, even if the jacket is only worth $100 in the first place. This bias can also affect salary negotiations, pricing decisions, and judgments about quality. Being aware of anchoring bias means questioning initial numbers or ideas and considering other possibilities before making a decision.

The bandwagon effect is the tendency to adopt beliefs or behaviors simply because many others do. This can be seen in trends, politics, and social media, where people follow popular opinions without critically evaluating them. For example, if a large group of people start investing in a certain stock, others may rush to do the same without researching whether it's a sound investment. Avoiding the bandwagon effect involves thinking independently and making choices based on facts rather than popularity.

Negativity bias makes people focus more on negative experiences than positive ones. This is why one bad review can seem more important than ten good ones or why people dwell on criticism longer than praise. This bias developed as a survival mechanism to help humans avoid danger, but in modern life, it can lead to unnecessary stress and anxiety. Practicing gratitude, looking at the bigger picture, and consciously focusing on positive experiences can help balance this tendency and create a healthier mindset.

Mirror image bias is when people assume that others, especially those from different groups or cultures, think and act just like they do. It's like looking in a mirror and expecting to see the same thoughts, values, and reasoning reflected back. This can lead to misunderstandings, as people may misinterpret the intentions or decisions of others based on their own beliefs rather than trying to see things from a different perspective. For example, in conflicts or negotiations, one side might assume that the other side shares the same motivations or fears, which can create tension and miscommunication. Overcoming mirror image bias requires awareness and the ability to step outside of one's own perspective to understand different viewpoints more accurately.

To work on mirror image bias, start by making a conscious effort to listen and observe without jumping to conclusions. When interacting with people from different backgrounds or perspectives, try to understand their motivations rather than assuming they think like you. Ask questions and stay curious instead of making assumptions. Reading about different cultures, histories, and viewpoints can also help expand your perspective. Practice empathy by putting yourself in someone else's shoes and considering how their experiences shape their thinking. If you find yourself assuming that someone else must see a situation the same way you do, take a step back and ask yourself if you might be overlooking key differences. Finally, be open to changing your mind when presented with new information. The more you challenge your own assumptions, the easier it becomes to see things from multiple perspectives.

Here are some examples of **negative beliefs and belief patterns** to use as a cheat sheet so you can start to have awareness and discernment about the rational truth of these statements and irrational fears from them:
- About oneself: "I am not good enough," "I am unlovable," "I am worthless," "I am inadequate," "I am a failure," "I am a burden," "I am too much," "I don't fit in," "I have to be perfect," "I am a fraud."
- About other people: "People will hurt me," "People are malicious," "People cannot be trusted."
- About the world: "The world is dangerous," "The world is unfair," "The world is scary."

Other negative beliefs to start changing:
- I don't deserve love.
- I am a bad person.
- I am terrible.
- I am worthless (inadequate).
- I am shameful.

- I am not lovable.
- I am a failure.
- I am unimportant.
- I am unworthy of happiness.
- I am undeserving of success.
- I am inherently flawed.
- I am untrustworthy.
- I am incapable of change.
- I am fundamentally broken.
- I don't belong.
- I am not good enough.
- I will never be happy.
- I am incapable.
- I am stupid.
- I am a burden to others.
- I am uninteresting.
- I am destined to be alone.
- I am undeserving of forgiveness.
- I am not in control.
- I am powerless (helpless).
- I am weak.
- I cannot get what I want.
- I am a failure (will fail).
- I cannot succeed.
- I have to be perfect (please everyone).
- I cannot stand it.
- I am inadequate.
- I cannot trust anyone.

Positive beliefs to start believing:
- I am capable and competent. Believing in your abilities and skills to handle tasks and challenges.
- I deserve love and happiness. Recognizing your inherent worth and right to experience joy and love.
- I can handle whatever comes my way. Trusting in your resilience

and adaptability to face difficulties. Every challenge is an opportunity to grow. Viewing obstacles as chances for personal development and learning.
- I am in control of my thoughts and emotions. Acknowledging your power to choose how you respond to situations.
- I am grateful for the good things in my life. Focusing on gratitude and appreciating the positive aspects of your life.
- I am worthy of success and abundance. Believing that you deserve to achieve your goals and enjoy prosperity.
- I trust myself and my decisions. Having confidence in your judgment and choices.
- I am a valuable and important person. Recognizing your unique contributions and significance.
- I learn from my mistakes and move forward. Accepting errors as part of the learning process and not dwelling on them.
- I am connected to others and not alone. Feeling a sense of belonging and support from relationships and community.
- I am creative and resourceful. Believing in your ability to find solutions and innovate.
- I am healthy and take care of my body. Valuing and prioritizing your physical well-being.
- I am kind and compassionate to myself and others. Practicing self-compassion and empathy towards others.
- I can make a positive difference in the world. Believing in your capacity to impact others and contribute to a better world.

This may sound mundane or insignificant, but just having a conversation with yourself either out loud or silently, can make huge differences in your transformation and understanding. After doing this for years I literally start to feel a shift in my body and my brain when talking things out loud.

Let's talk a little more about PTSD shall we? I'm writing about this a lot for a reason. We need to read and hear things many times before we can grasp it fully.

Post Traumatic Stress Disorder (PTSD) means you've had one or more traumatic experiences in the past and your body still carries with it the fearfulness or trauma from the experiences.

After the trauma happened to you, there can be triggers in the NOW moment that can activate that stress response, creating an onslaught of uncomfortable sensations and experiences. The most popular triggers are loud fireworks and other similar noises that can trigger a war veteran and activate PTSD from wartime. So, their bodies and minds think that it's gunfire from war but it's just fireworks. That right there is what we are working on to rewiring so that the body doesn't get triggered into a panic event.

Physioneurosis is chronic PTSD, a mental disorder with both physiological and psychological components where mental or emotional stress manifests as physical symptoms in the body. This condition is also known as psychosomatic disorder. With this, bodies continue to re-experience the frightening and terrible situations, and the event keeps coming back in terms of images, behaviors and physical sensations. Another way to explain physioneurosis is that it refers to physical symptoms that arise from psychological or emotional stress rather than from a direct physical cause. Trauma is actually (and unfortunately) very common, outside of what the average person would think:

- One in five women have had sexual molestation – many men too.
- One of four kids is beaten and, or abused.
- One in eight kids see physical fights between their parents.

IMPORTANT NOTE:
It's important to remember that nothing affects everyone in exactly the same way. I want to emphasize that again. Factors like physical pain—especially in today's world of ultra–processed foods, sedentary habits, and chronic stress—can stem from deeper issues like autoimmunity and gut dysbiosis. These imbalances often

lead to body–wide inflammation, which can drive a wide range of diseases, disorders, and persistent physical pain. Everyone's path and response are unique, but these modern influences are worth examining closely.

Examples of Physioneurosis:
- Stomach Aches and Ulcers:
    - **Scenario:** A person is going through a highly stressful period at work with constant deadlines and pressure from their boss.
    - **Symptom:** They start experiencing frequent stomach aches and, over time, develop a stomach ulcer.
    - **Explanation:** The stress and anxiety from work are causing physical reactions in the body, leading to digestive issues.
- Headaches and Migraines:
    - **Scenario:** An individual is dealing with significant personal problems, such as a breakup or family conflict.
    - **Symptom:** They begin to suffer from chronic headaches or migraines.
    - **Explanation:** Emotional distress triggers tension and changes in blood flow to the brain, causing headaches.
- Back Pain:
    - **Scenario:** Someone is feeling overwhelmed by financial troubles and the uncertainty of their future.
    - **Symptom:** They start having severe lower back pain without any obvious physical injury.
    - **Explanation:** The psychological stress is causing muscle tension and pain in the back.
- Chest Pain:
    - **Scenario:** A person is experiencing intense anxiety about their health, constantly worrying about serious illnesses.
    - **Symptom:** They feel chest pain and tightness.
    - **Explanation:** Anxiety can lead to chest pain due to increased muscle tension and heart rate, mimicking symptoms of a heart condition.

- Irritable Bowel Syndrome (IBS):
    - **Scenario:** A student is anxious about their exams and future prospects.
    - **Symptom:** They develop symptoms of IBS, such as frequent diarrhea or constipation.
    - **Explanation:** Stress and anxiety can disrupt normal digestive processes, leading to IBS.

How Physioneurosis Occurs:

When a person experiences stress, the body reacts by releasing stress hormones like cortisol and adrenaline, which prepare the body to deal with the stressor by increasing heart rate, muscle tension, and energy supplies. If the stress is chronic, the continuous release of these hormones can lead to physical symptoms, such as constant muscle tension causing pain and changes in digestive function resulting in gastrointestinal issues. The mind and body are interconnected, meaning that emotional and mental states can significantly impact physical health, which explains why emotional stress can result in physical symptoms.

Managing stress effectively involves a combination of techniques such as mindfulness, meditation, and deep breathing exercises, which can help reduce stress and its physical manifestations.

Cognitive–behavioral therapy (CBT) and other forms of psychotherapy are also beneficial, as they aid individuals in managing stress and anxiety, thereby reducing the likelihood of physical symptoms. Additionally, maintaining a healthy lifestyle through regular exercise, a balanced diet, and adequate sleep can improve overall well–being and make it easier to cope with stress. It's also important to consult healthcare providers to rule out any underlying physical conditions and to receive appropriate treatment for both physical and psychological symptoms.

I'm going to reiterate here again in different words so that you can keep hearing this over and over again.

Reacting to mild stressors as if your life is in danger, such as hyperreactivity and road rage, can be traced back to trauma's profound impact on our senses and brain. When trauma occurs, it assaults all of our senses—ears, skin, eyes—sending distress signals deep into our primitive amygdala, the brain's fear center. The amygdala interprets these signals as either safe or dangerous, triggering the fight, flight, or freeze/collapse responses. This overactivation can lead individuals to react disproportionately to minor stressors, behaving as if they are in imminent danger. Understanding this connection highlights the importance of addressing trauma to mitigate these hyperreactive behaviors and improve emotional regulation.

Exposure Therapy

Let's talk about a very important type of therapy called Exposure Therapy. I've used this a lot in my life, and it has helped me so much because I'm the type of person and my body is a certain way that allows this to work better for me. I don't like to be thrown in with the wolves so to speak and just have rapid change or to transform in that way. I need the gradual shift that this brings.

Exposure Therapy is a type of treatment often used to help people with anxiety disorders, including PTSD. This therapy involves gradually and systematically exposing individuals to the situations, objects, or thoughts that trigger their anxiety. The main goal is to reduce the fear and avoidance behavior associated with these triggers, making the person more comfortable and less anxious over time.

Gradual Exposure: this starts with exposing the person to less anxiety–provoking situations and then gradually moving towards more challenging ones. This method often uses a hierarchy, or list, of feared stimuli, starting from the least to the most frightening.

Desensitization: this is gradual exposure to the anxiety source. It helps to reduce the physical symptoms of anxiety while facing the fear. As you are gradually confronting your fear, you can use any therapy we talk about to manage your fear.

In Vivo Exposure: this means directly confronting the feared object or situation in real life. For example, someone afraid of dogs might gradually start by looking at pictures of dogs, then visiting a place where there are dogs, and eventually petting a dog.

Image Exposure: When direct confrontation isn't possible, the person vividly imagines the feared object or situation. This can help them process and reduce their fear.

Interoceptive Exposure: This involves deliberately inducing physical sensations that are harmless but often feared, like an increased heart rate, to help the person learn that these sensations are not dangerous.

Exposure therapy helps individuals by gradually reducing fear and anxiety responses, allowing them to handle anxiety without avoiding the situation. This process increases control over thoughts and feelings, as repeated exposure changes how they think about and react to the feared situation. It also enhances their ability to tolerate distressing situations, making them less sensitive to anxiety–provoking stimuli over time. As a result, their overall functioning and quality of life improve, enabling them to engage more fully in daily activities.

Exposure therapy is effective for various conditions, including PTSD, where it helps individuals confront and process traumatic memories and phobias, by addressing specific fears like flying or heights; social anxiety, by easing fears related to social interactions and OCD, by reducing compulsive behaviors through facing anxiety–provoking thoughts and situations.

Research strongly supports the effectiveness of exposure therapy for treating anxiety disorders and PTSD, with studies showing significant improvements in symptoms and overall functioning for those who undergo this type of therapy.

Other Therapies to Use Alongside Exposure Therapy:

Cognitive Behavioral Therapy (CBT): CBT focuses on identifying and challenging irrational thoughts and beliefs. When combined with exposure therapy, it can help individuals reframe their thinking about the feared object or situation, making the exposure more effective.

Mindfulness–Based Stress Reduction (MBSR): MBSR teaches mindfulness techniques to stay present and reduce anxiety. This can be particularly useful during exposure therapy, as it helps individuals manage their anxiety responses in real time. Journaling with this would be great as well.

Systematic Desensitization: This technique combines gradual exposure with relaxation exercises. By teaching individuals to relax while facing their fears, it can help reduce the anxiety associated with exposure.

Acceptance and Commitment Therapy (ACT): ACT encourages individuals to accept their thoughts and feelings rather than fight them, while committing to behavior changes aligned with their values. This can complement exposure therapy by helping individuals tolerate the discomfort associated with exposure.

Some examples of exposure therapy and what you can do:

Managing Social Anxiety
Gradual Exposure: begin by imagining social interactions. Then, progress to saying hello to strangers, having brief conversations, attending small gatherings, and finally participating in larger social events.

Combining with Mindfulness–Based Stress Reduction (MBSR) Mindfulness techniques can help the person stay present and reduce anxiety during social interactions. They learn to observe their thoughts without judgment and remain calm.

Overcoming a Fear of Dogs

Gradual Exposure: Start by looking at pictures of dogs. Next, watch videos of dogs, observe a dog from a distance, be in the same room as a calm dog, and eventually pet a dog.

Combining with Systematic Desensitization: This approach might involve teaching the person relaxation/vagus nerve techniques, such as deep breathing or progressive muscle relaxation, to use when exposed to dogs as long as the situation is rationally and logically SAFE. This helps them associate the presence of dogs with a state of calm rather than anxiety.

Coping with PTSD

Image Exposure: The individual vividly imagines the traumatic event in a safe and controlled environment, repeatedly describing it in detail to reduce its emotional impact over time.

Combining with Eye Movement Desensitization and Reprocessing
(EMDR) involves recalling traumatic memories while performing guided eye movements. This can help process and reduce the distress associated with the memories.

IMPORATANT NOTE:
EMDR NEEDS to be done with a professional. I've never done EMDR, but it is a popular approach. The research I've done is here for you to contemplate.

Let's recap, so when you are in a situation where you are confronting your fear only very slightly, you will have to find where the line is. You will have to approach your fear to find out where to start. Once you find that, you should already have some therapies you will use. For example, as you approach very slightly this fear, you can stop and start journaling like we talk about earlier in the chapter. Just see if any symptoms and sensations diminish. After journaling you can try some vagus nerve techniques that we also went over. Balloon breathing, ear massage, cold therapy and so on!

If you feel overwhelmed at the start, maybe you went too far and need to back up a bit. OR you can try the EFT technique, tapping for panic. Once that calms you a bit then you can go into the other therapies. This was my approach for years and it really is one of the biggest pieces that helped my recovery. You could try some yoga, exercise or Qigong that we'll go into in the next 3 chapters. I hope this is starting become more and more clear in your mind. There is so much help out there! I really like Dr. Dawn-Elise Snipes, she has a PhD in Counseling and is a family therapist. Here's a snippet of some of her work with trauma, PTSD, and C-PTSD.

We have what's called the orienting reflex. This is a function of every organism and it's a response or reflex of any external stimuli. As babies, the vagus nerve takes in stimuli and reports it to the brain and the brain consults the schema and it says, "is this information happy, fear or pain?" Schema is our brain's filing system. The vagus nerve and the brain, interpret information and file it into organized information. This is to keep us safe in survival situations and to allow us to be prepared when we receive similar information from the past and to better interpret information in the moment. For example, someone's brain might have a file folder that is labeled, "hot stove top, don't touch!" Or something irrational, "My ex broke my heart, everyone will end up breaking my heart."

In psychology, a schema is a mental model that the brain uses to organize information about the world, and to help people interpret new experiences. Schemas are built from memories of unique experiences and can be influenced by a person's self–knowledge and cultural background. They can help people think and learn new information quickly, but they can also make it difficult to retain information that doesn't fit with existing beliefs.

People with complex PTSD (C–PTSD), anxiety, or borderline personality disorder are at a higher risk of poor vagal tone, due to the close connection between the vagus nerve and the amygdala, the brain's fear and survival center. This connection keeps the hypothalamic–pituitary–adrenal (HPA) axis and the orienting reflex in a state of high alert, contributing to hypervigilance.

Over time, chronic activation of the stress response can shrink the hippocampus, the area of the brain crucial for emotional regulation and memory. This not only makes it harder to manage emotions but also contributes to cognitive challenges. Additionally, prolonged stress wears down receptor cells, leaving them fatigued and less responsive—essentially "numb," which further disrupts proper brain and body function. The more often you're stuck in fight–or–flight mode, the more nutrients your body burns through just to keep up. In today's world, where nutrient deficiencies are already common due to processed diets and chronic stress, this has become a serious compounding issue that can spiral into deeper dysfunction. Not to mention, lack of blood flow to the brain when in this hypervigilant state.

The Default Mode Network (DMN) refers to the part of our brain that operates on autopilot, managing automatic thoughts and trigger responses. When negative, PTSD related triggered responses dominate, they reinforce the connection to the amygdala—the brain's fear center—while also reducing vagal tone. This makes it increasingly difficult to turn off the fear response.

To counteract this, you need to override the default mode by engaging in exercises and techniques provided in this book. These include using the logical brain before the emotional brain takes over, through practices like journaling, Socratic questioning, mindfulness, meditation, and ritual practices. Additionally, actions such as changing diet and nutrition, increasing awareness and altering automatic thoughts, positive self–talk therapy, and professional talk therapy can be beneficial. Techniques specifically aimed at stimulating the vagus nerve by gargling, humming, singing, neck massage, stretching, and the Valsalva maneuver, also play a crucial role. Other practices include HRV biofeedback, smiling, laughter, desensitization exercises, CBT, yoga, deep breathing, Qigong, and martial arts.

I'm reiterating this information throughout the book intentionally. I present it in various ways and through different experts so that the concepts become familiar and ingrained. Our brains often need to encounter information multiple times—sometimes 7 to 8 times—before it fully sinks in or is stored in long-term memory.

We are constantly making decisions about what to pay attention to, as our senses—sight, hearing, smell, taste, and touch—send information to the brain via the vagus nerve. The brain then consults our mental schemas and "file folders" to interpret this information, determining whether it signals fear, happiness, pain, or other emotions. If the incoming information is familiar, the vagus nerve guides the brain on how to respond appropriately. However, if the information is unknown, intense, or unexpected, it triggers the orienting response, alerting the body to potential danger.

When the fear mode is activated, the Default Mode Network (DMN) can take over, making it harder to process information rationally. Basically, it's your primal brainstem, lizard brain, taking over. Sights, sounds, and smells associated with the fearful experience can become linked with danger, causing the individual to perceive threats more frequently. Strengthening the parasympathetic vagal response, which promotes calmness and safety, begins with creating safe environments and recognizing faulty expectations or schemas.

Gradual reconditioning through exposure to stimuli and intentional responses can weaken the connection between the (DMN) and the amygdala (which is what we want). This process enhances the activation of the parasympathetic response, helping to "reprogram" the Hypothalamic Pituitary – Adrenal (HPA) axis, reducing dysregulation and inflammation in the body.

Are you in a state of safety, activation, where you feel calm and secure, or in mobilization, where your body is preparing to respond to a perceived threat? How you respond to these stimuli can change the perception of anxiety.

Next, I want to again share these vagus nerve stimulators, they are very popular right now and for a very good reason. So many people of all ages are so stressed and their bodies and nervous systems are being overloaded with stimulation. How ironic to use a stimulator to calm you down from over stimulation!

First device I'll include is the Apollo neuro. This goes around the wrist like a watch. My wife has this one, she loves it. This is not specifically stimulating the vagus nerve but it's like giving your body a nice hug with gentle vibrations and frequencies.

Next is the Verelief products by Hoolest. My wife has the Verelief pro headset version and it's working for her. I personally haven't used them yet, because I have or had a unique condition where I had brady–tachycardia, where my heart beats too fast and then too slow. My cardiologist doesn't want me to use them or only do it very minimally and on one side at a time, and not at night when my heart rate drops to below 50. It's better than it used to be and I'm doing very well, which is why I'm writing this book.

Pulsetto is another device to look into. There are loads of great YouTube videos reviewing these products in real time and over periods of time to get a good idea about them. That's what I did before purchasing. There are many other devices but from these you can find what best suits you.

Along with devices, I want to share with you an app called WellTory that has helped me and is very important for general information about heart rate variability. It provides detailed information about the heart and nervous system. You need a smart watch of some kind or a smart phone. You can get the basics for free and can use it one time a day. I subscribe monthly so I can use it multiple times a day. If you have health issues and/or are maybe a little older like me, I think it's important to have.

Psychology – Key Concepts

Here I want to introduce you to some basics in modern psychology related to different areas of thought. If something catches your attention, you can find a library of information on any one of these topics.

Psychology introduces foundational concepts that help us understand human behavior, thought processes, and emotions. One of the most significant debates in psychology is the nature versus nurture argument, which examines the extent to which our genes (nature) or our environment (nurture) shape who we are. This debate addresses questions like whether intelligence is inherited or developed, or if personality traits are something we're born with or learn over time. Today, most psychologists agree that both genetics and environment interact to shape an individual's behavior and personality. For instance, someone may have a genetic predisposition toward a particular trait, such as anxiety, but whether they experience it can depend on their life experiences and environment.

Another key topic is developmental psychology, which studies how people grow and change throughout their lives, from infancy to old age. Psychologists like Jean Piaget and Erik Erikson developed theories on stages of development that describe how children and adults progress through different cognitive, social, and emotional stages. Piaget's stages of cognitive development, for example, outline how children develop logical thinking abilities as they age, moving from concrete to abstract thinking. Erikson's stages of psychosocial development describe challenges we face at each stage of life, such as developing trust as infants or identity during adolescence.

In understanding behavior, psychologists explore different psychological perspectives. The biological perspective focuses on how the brain, nervous system, and genetic makeup influence our actions and emotions. The behavioral perspective, developed by pioneers like John Watson and B.F. Skinner, emphasizes the role of learning and environment. Behavioral psychologists argue that we learn behaviors through reinforcement and punishment, shaping our actions based on what brings positive or negative outcomes. The cognitive perspective examines how we think, remember, and process information, emphasizing how our thoughts influence our behavior. The humanistic perspective, championed by psychologists like Carl Rogers and Abraham Maslow, suggests that people are inherently good and motivated to achieve their full potential, with a focus on personal growth and self-actualization.

Examining mental health disorders provides a basic understanding of conditions like depression, anxiety, bipolar disorder, and schizophrenia. Students learn how these disorders are diagnosed and the various approaches to treatment, including therapy and medication. Therapeutic approaches include cognitive–behavioral therapy (CBT), which aims to change negative thought patterns, and psychodynamic therapy, which explores unconscious thoughts and feelings. Each approach is rooted in different psychological perspectives and offers unique methods for addressing mental health issues.

Another critical topic is social psychology, which examines how people influence and are influenced by others. Social psychologists study concepts like conformity, obedience, and group dynamics to understand why people behave differently in groups or follow social norms. Classic experiments, such as Stanley Milgram's obedience study and Philip Zimbardo's Stanford prison experiment, demonstrate the powerful impact of authority and social roles on behavior, shedding light on how individuals can act in ways they might not otherwise when under pressure.

Finally, psychology explores research methods used to study the mind and behavior. Psychologists rely on various methods, including experiments, surveys, case studies, and naturalistic observation, to gather data and draw conclusions. These methods allow researchers to test hypotheses, understand relationships between variables, and build a scientific understanding of psychological phenomena. Learning about research ethics is also crucial, as psychologists must ensure the well–being of their participants, maintain confidentiality, and conduct studies responsibly.

In summary, introductory psychology provides a broad overview of the many factors that influence human behavior and mental processes. By examining concepts like nature versus nurture, stages of development, different psychological perspectives, mental health disorders, social psychology, and research methods, students gain a foundational understanding of the complexities of the human mind. This knowledge sets the stage for further exploration in psychology, whether one is interested in clinical practice, research, or simply understanding more about human behavior.

Control Issues and Expectations

Trying to control every aspect of your life with an iron grip will likely lead to overwhelming stress for both you and those around you, causing unnecessary anxiety. Hopefully, by this point in the book, you've gained some skills and techniques to help you let go of this need for control and embrace a more flexible, go–with–the–flow approach, when appropriate, of course.

Unchecked expectations can be a major source of stress, often leading to disappointment when reality doesn't align with the ideal outcomes we set in our minds. By placing impossible demands on ourselves, we're essentially setting ourselves up for failure and frustration. This is where cognitive distortions come into play. For example, thinking, "If I don't work 24 hours a day, I'm worthless and a disappointment to my parents, my boss, and myself," is a classic case of all–or–nothing thinking and unrealistic expectations. Believing that we must meet such extreme standards to feel worthy or valuable can lead to chronic stress, self–doubt, and a constant fear of failure.

Learning to manage and adjust expectations is key to reducing anxiety. Embracing realistic goals and allowing yourself to do your best within reasonable limits can create a healthier mindset, one that accepts progress over perfection. By loosening the grip of control and cultivating balanced expectations, you'll not only reduce your stress but also find a greater sense of peace and fulfillment.

BRINGING IT ALL TOGETHER (AGAIN):

The root cause of PTSD and anxiety is both complex and layered, involving the brain, body, thoughts, and environment. These are all intricately connected. One of the biggest misconceptions is that PTSD is just about "bad memories" or negative thinking patterns ABOUT past events. In reality, it is a physiological, neurological, and emotional imprint left by overwhelming or unresolved trauma. The root of PTSD lies not just in what happened, but in how the brain and body responded to what happened—and how they were unable to fully process or recover from it.

At the core of PTSD is a **dysregulated nervous system**. When a person experiences trauma, especially overwhelming or inescapable stress, the brain's survival systems kick in—particularly the amygdala (which detects threats) and the hypothalamic–pituitary–adrenal (HPA) axis, which releases stress hormones like cortisol and adrenaline. If the event is too intense to process, this system can get stuck on "high alert." Even long after the trauma has passed, the brain and body act as if the danger is still present. By the way, a dysregulated nervous system, means a dysregulated immune system, digestive system and life.

So, when a trigger appears—like fireworks for a combat veteran—it may not be the conscious thought ("that sounds like gunfire") that sets off the reaction. Instead, it's often the sensory input—the sound, smell, or body sensation—that bypasses conscious thought entirely and instantly activates the limbic system. This is why PTSD symptoms can arise even when someone knows rationally that they're safe: the body remembers, even when the mind tries to forget. Remember the limbic system is the emotional and memory/learning center that bypasses the logical thinking brain and triggers your emotional center. That's not what we want in cases like this, where there are irrational fears and situations.

That said, thoughts do play a role. Once the nervous system is activated, the mind tries to make sense of the alarm, often looping into fearful thoughts or catastrophic interpretations, which feed the stress response further. This creates feedback looping where the body triggers the mind, the mind triggers the body, and the cycle continues. The HPA axis remains overactive, inflammation rises, digestion slows, sleep is disturbed, and the body becomes worn down over time.

So, what needs to be healed first: the stored trauma in the brain, or the stress fire in the body?

The honest answer is both. You need to "put out the fire" in the body—calm the overactive stress response, regulate the nervous system, and rebuild safety in the physical self. This may involve somatic therapies, (yoga, bodywork, etc.) breathing techniques, vagus nerve activation, grounding practices, nutrition, rest, and possibly more. But you also need to address the root in the brain—the unprocessed trauma, the stuck memory, or the meaning your subconscious has attached to the event. That's where therapy, trauma processing, and techniques in this book can come in.

Healing PTSD is not **just** about "changing your thoughts," nor is it only about "relaxing the body." It's about restoring the connection between body and mind and helping both realize **YOU ARE SAFE NOW**. Only then can the trauma be fully released, not just intellectually, but physiologically as well. Healing is not about forgetting what happened but helping the body and brain stop reliving it.

Let's talk a little about the highly important thyroid here. This might seem out of place, but it's just a reminder to how important it is and how it can affect our psychology and cognitive function.

The thyroid is a small, butterfly–shaped gland in the front of your neck that plays a big role in your health. It controls your metabolism, energy levels, temperature regulation, and even your mood by releasing hormones like T3 and T4. When you're dealing with

PTSD or chronic illness, the thyroid can become imbalanced—either slowing down (hypothyroid) or becoming overactive/disbalanced (hyperthyroid)—due to long-term stress on the body.

Chronic stress and trauma increase cortisol and adrenaline, which can interfere with how the thyroid works, leading to symptoms like fatigue, weight changes, brain fog, anxiety, depression, and digestive problems. The thyroid and adrenal glands are deeply connected, so when one is off, the other often struggles too. Supporting thyroid health means managing stress, eating enough nutrients like iodine, selenium, zinc, and B vitamins, and healing and balancing the nervous system. When the thyroid is supported, it becomes easier to feel emotionally stable, have energy, and recover from long-term illness.

When our stress system (called the HPA – Hypothalamus Pituitary Adrenal axis) has been out of balance for a long time—whether from trauma, chronic illness, anxiety, or emotional burnout—it can quietly slow down your thyroid, even if the thyroid gland itself is technically healthy on paper or on blood testing. High stress leads to chronically elevated cortisol, and cortisol sends signals to your body to slow down in order to conserve energy. One of the first systems to respond is your thyroid. The thyroid mostly produces a hormone called T4, but your body has to convert that into T3, the active form that actually powers your metabolism, brain function, and energy levels. Chronic stress interferes with this conversion, sometimes creating a form called 'reverse T3,' which blocks your cells from using thyroid hormone effectively, even when your blood tests appear "normal."

Stress can also reduce TSH, the signal your brain sends to the thyroid to tell it how much hormone to make. If your brain is burned out or overwhelmed, that signal weakens, and your thyroid slows down in response. On top of that, stress damages your gut and liver—the two main places where T4 is converted into active T3. Over time, this disruption can even trigger autoimmune reactions against your thyroid, especially in people with unresolved immune stress or gut issues.

If this pattern has been active for years, you may feel tired all the time, mentally foggy, emotionally unstable, cold in your hands and feet, or stuck in a body that won't respond to healthy changes. The good news is that this can be reversed. When you start supporting your stress system through better sleep, gentle movement, nutrient support, and nervous system regulation, the thyroid often begins to recover too. Healing the HPA axis is not separate from healing the thyroid; in truth, they are deeply connected parts of the same system. Everything in this book is geared towards healing the HPA axis, thyroid and not to mention many, many other chronic health problems.

Takeaways from Chapter 7

- Cognitive Distortions – read through them and begin to recognize how they're showing up in your life—and in others' lives, too. Awareness is the first step toward change.
- Automatic Thoughts – start noticing the thoughts that pop into your mind throughout the day. Reflect on them, write them down, and don't be afraid to question them!
- Socratic Questioning – use this method to dig deeper into those automatic thoughts. Ask yourself: "Is this thought really true?" "What's the evidence?" "Is there another way to look at this?"
- ABCDE of Cognitive Behavioral Therapy – begin connecting the dots between the Activating event, your Beliefs, and the Consequences. Most people skip over the Belief part, but that's where the real insight happens.
- Vagus Nerve Stimulators and Devices – these can be useful tools to support nervous system regulation. Just make sure to do your own research and use them safely.
- Exposure Therapy – take it slow. Pace yourself. This can be one of the hardest, yet most effective, tools to work through fear and avoidance.
- Journaling – a powerful way to organize your thoughts and shift from the emotional brain to the **logical, rational brain.** When managing anxiety, PTSD, or stress, this is where we want to operate most of the time.
- The Reality of Life – sometimes, life is just hard and accepting that can be oddly empowering. Not everything needs fixing, but for what can be improved, real change is possible. Life doesn't have to be as hard as it feels.
- Values–Based Living – in your meditations and reflections, shift focus toward meaningful values like health, family, relationships, exercise, and purpose–driven work. These anchor you when things get shaky.

- Psychology 101 – learn the basics. Understanding the fundamentals of how the mind works is a huge asset in any healing or personal growth journey.
- Letting Go of Control – surrender a bit. Embrace flow. Avoid setting yourself up for failure with rigid expectations. Flexibility leads to more peace, less pressure.

Here are a few Cognitive Behavior Journal templates for you to practice (if you're reading this digitally, then just copy this onto paper or into a separate file):

CBT Journal Template

Date: _____

Time of Entry: _____

1. Situation: What happened? Where were you? Who were you with?
_____
_____
_____

2. Automatic Thoughts: What thoughts or beliefs immediately came up? Be honest and specific.
_____
_____
_____

3. Emotions / Feelings: What emotions did you feel? Rate intensity from 0–100%. Example: Anxiety – 80%, Anger – 60%
_____
_____
_____

4. Physical Sensations: What did you notice in your body (tight chest, clenched jaw, etc.)?
_____
_____
_____
_____

5. Behaviors / Reactions: What did you do or not do in response to the situation or emotions?

_____
_____
_____
_____

6. Thinking Errors / Cognitive Distortions: Did you notice any unhelpful thinking patterns (e.g. catastrophizing, mind reading, black–and–white thinking)?

_____
_____
_____
_____

7. Evidence For and Against the Thought:
— Evidence for:

_____
_____
_____
_____

— Evidence against:

_____
_____
_____
_____

8. Balanced Thought / Reframe: What would be a more realistic or helpful way to look at the situation?

_____
_____
_____

9. New Emotions: After reframing, what do you feel now? Rate intensity from 0–100%

_____
_____

10. What Will I Do Differently Next Time? What healthy action, boundary, or self–talk could help next time?

CBT Journal Template

Date: _____

Time of Entry: _____

1. Situation: What happened? Where were you? Who were you with?

2. Automatic Thoughts: What thoughts or beliefs immediately came up? Be honest and specific.

3. Emotions / Feelings: What emotions did you feel? Rate intensity from 0–100%. Example: Anxiety – 80%, Anger – 60%

4. Physical Sensations: What did you notice in your body (tight chest, clenched jaw, etc.)?

___

5. Behaviors / Reactions: What did you do or not do in response to the situation or emotions?

___

6. Thinking Errors / Cognitive Distortions: Did you notice any unhelpful thinking patterns (e.g. catastrophizing, mind reading, black–and–white thinking)?

___

7. Evidence For and Against the Thought:
— Evidence for:

___

— Evidence against:

___

8. Balanced Thought / Reframe: What would be a more realistic or helpful way to look at the situation?

___

9. New Emotions: After reframing, what do you feel now? Rate intensity from 0–100%

_____
_____
_____

10. What Will I Do Differently Next Time? What healthy action, boundary, or self–talk could help next time?

_____
_____
_____
_____

CBT Journal Template

Date: _____

Time of Entry: _____

1. Situation: What happened? Where were you? Who were you with?

_____
_____
_____

2. Automatic Thoughts: What thoughts or beliefs immediately came up? Be honest and specific.

_____
_____
_____
_____

3. Emotions / Feelings: What emotions did you feel? Rate intensity from 0–100%. Example: Anxiety – 80%, Anger – 60%

_____
_____
_____
_____

4. Physical Sensations: What did you notice in your body (tight chest, clenched jaw, etc.)?

_____
_____
_____
_____

5. Behaviors / Reactions: What did you do or not do in response to the situation or emotions?

_____
_____
_____
_____

6. Thinking Errors / Cognitive Distortions: Did you notice any unhelpful thinking patterns (e.g. catastrophizing, mind reading, black–and–white thinking)?

_____
_____
_____
_____

7. Evidence For and Against the Thought:
– Evidence for:

_____
_____
_____
_____

– Evidence against:

_____
_____

8. Balanced Thought / Reframe: What would be a more realistic or helpful way to look at the situation?

_____
_____
_____

9. New Emotions: After reframing, what do you feel now? Rate intensity from 0–100%

_____
_____
_____

10. What Will I Do Differently Next Time? What healthy action, boundary, or self–talk could help next time?

_____
_____
_____
_____

Chapter 8
Yoga – Rise Up and Out of Your Shell

"The happiness of your life depends upon the quality of your thoughts."
— *Marcus Aurelius*

In this chapter, my goal isn't to teach you specific yoga poses or guide you through a full sequence. Instead, I want to provide you with the knowledge and awareness of yoga's benefits and how you can integrate them into your daily life. I want to share the foundational wisdom and understanding of yoga—some basics, key concepts, and a few simple exercises and techniques. More than anything, I hope to inspire you to explore yoga in a way that feels natural and meaningful in your daily life.

For actual instruction, there are countless yoga videos on YouTube and studios you can explore, and I highly recommend checking them out. Maybe by the time you're reading this, I'll have added more yoga flows to my own YouTube channel @WasenshiDo. For now, my primary focus is on teaching martial arts, though I do have some yoga videos on the channel. For beginner to intermediate yoga, I highly recommend Yoga with Adriene on YouTube.

Let's get straight into it. Yoga, or "Yug" in ancient times, means "to Yoke," which basically means union. Yoga is the union between mind, body and spirit. If you're familiar with the slang, "get yoked," which a term bodybuilders use, then you know that means to get really connected with your mind and body! Joking aside, yoga has helped me tremendously in my life. Even just practicing Hatha yoga, which is just physical stretching and movements/ postures, can be greatly beneficial.

Yoga asana (the physical postures) allows more blood flow to the muscles, more nerve conduction and energy flow. Energy meridians can open and flow more freely, allowing better communication between the brain and organs. Yoga can also help the endocrine glands function better.

I've been practicing yoga since 2009 and received my 200–hour Yoga Teacher Certification in 2017. My goal here is to offer you a grounded, accessible approach to Yoga, something practical and down to earth that supports anxiety relief, stress reduction, and overall health and wellness. While some of the concepts might seem a bit "up in the clouds," the roots of this practice are deeply grounded. That's how I like to frame it. This book is based on what has helped me personally, helped others I've worked with, and draws from teachings that have stood the test of time for centuries.

We already covered breathing techniques in Chapter 5, so we won't dive too deeply into Pranayama here. Instead, I want to begin with the yoga of the mind, before moving into the body. In the next section, we'll talk about how applying mild, intentional stress through postures and breath can signal safety to the nervous system and create real calm in the body.

Eastern philosophy and yoga of the mind are deeply intertwined. Yoga is not just about relaxation, it's a pathway to self–awareness, emotional balance, and resilience.

Mindfulness and Introspection

Yoga encourages you to become present with yourself, which naturally leads to deeper self-reflection. This is incredibly helpful when it comes to managing emotions and navigating everyday stress. For some people, this kind of self–awareness can feel intense or overwhelming at first. If that's you, take it slow. Baby steps are not only okay, but they're also encouraged.

Stress, Anxiety, and PTSD Relief

If you often feel emotionally reactive, easily overwhelmed, or stuck in stress, yoga can help regulate your internal state. Chronic stress can wreak havoc on the body and mind, but yoga gives you tools to calm the nervous system. With time, you'll begin to notice when you're veering into stress and have the means to return to center. Breathing techniques and certain postures activate the vagus nerve (which we covered earlier), supporting emotional regulation and a greater sense of calm.

Mood Enhancement and Emotional Balance

Yoga also supports hormonal health and helps balance key neurotransmitters like serotonin and dopamine. These chemical messengers are essential to regulating mood, focus, and energy—and yoga can play a big role in keeping them in check.

The key to transformation is consistency. You have to show up for yourself. By slowing down your movements, deepening your breath, and engaging in stretching, twisting, and even light contortion, you increase circulation, regulate hormone levels, and activate the parasympathetic nervous system—all of which are linked to better vagus nerve activity. Better circulation means more oxygen and nutrients are delivered to your tissues, which leads to improved vitality and well-being over time.

To switch gears for a moment, here's a fun way to bring the elements into your lifestyle. This should help you view life from a fresh perspective and expand your mindset in new and exciting ways.

Earth Element: Grounding for Body, Mind, and Spirit

One of the first things I do upon waking is take a small pinch of unrefined salt—like Celtic Sea salt—with a glass of water. This simple ritual helps support hydration, mineral balance, and a sense of rootedness, and it aligns beautifully with the Earth element (plus I get the water element as well). Salt is a natural conductor and a fundamental building block of life, connecting us to the mineral–rich structure of the earth itself.

Walking barefoot outside, known as *Earthing* or *Grounding*, is another deeply nourishing Earth practice. It helps discharge built–up static electricity, balances the body's electrical field, and has been scientifically shown to reduce inflammation, regulate cortisol, and even improve sleep. It also strengthens posture and foot mechanics when done with care—especially when you're mindful of maintaining a proper arch and walking with intention. Grounding restores the body's connection to the natural world, something we've lost in the modern, rubber–soled, screen–saturated world.

When practicing Earthing, make sure to walk in clean, natural environments and steer clear of areas treated with pesticides, fertilizers, or heavy pollutants, especially in city or suburban settings. Also, be aware of potential parasites like hookworms or ticks that can enter through the soles of the feet. If you're immune–compromised or dealing with chronic illness, consider safer options like standing barefoot on rocks, untreated wood, or clean concrete.

Another overlooked Earth–related factor is your bed frame. If you're energy sensitive like I am, you may have noticed that sleeping on a metal frame can interfere with rest and energy levels. It's not just intuition—metal frames can act as antennas, amplifying EMF exposure from Wi-Fi, cell phones, and nearby electronics while you sleep. Consider switching to a natural wood bed frame, which doesn't conduct electricity and offers a more grounded sleep environment. Be cautious with plastic alternatives as well. While they may not carry EMFs, many off–gas harmful VOCs (volatile organic compounds), including bromine and flame retardants. These toxins can quietly affect hormone health, especially the thyroid, and contribute to sleep disturbances, anxiety, and immune dysfunction over time.

The Earth element reminds us to slow down, stay grounded, and reconnect to nature in real and practical ways. It's about simplifying, strengthening the foundation—both physically and mentally—and finding stillness in a fast-moving world.

Another mental and emotional principle worth reflecting on is finding the right balance between mental toughness, inner firmness, and stubbornness. While it's important to stand your ground and remain emotionally resilient, leaning too far into stubbornness can become rigid and limiting. On the emotional side, think of it as having strength and composure without being overly guarded. If your defenses are always up, you may be cutting yourself off from connection and growth. On the flip side, being too open, overly trusting, or highly reactive may signal a lack of grounding—too much fire, not enough Earth.

Emotional overwhelm and volatility are often signs of a dysregulated nervous system in need of stability, calm, and grounding practices to restore balance. The goal is to cultivate strong roots without building walls. Our physical bodies are associated with the Earth element, so here's to keeping our body as healthy as possible.

Whether it's with your first glass of water, your bare feet in the grass, or the surface you sleep on each night, anchoring yourself to Earth brings calm, clarity, and resilience.

Water – Hydration for Vitality and Flow

Hydration is one of the most foundational yet overlooked elements of health and it aligns perfectly with the Water element, which represents flow, nourishment, and adaptability. Personally, I drink Dr. Berg's electrolyte powder daily to ensure proper mineral balance, and I always opt for natural spring water whenever possible. For a long time, we had clean, mineral-rich five-gallon spring water delivered to our home. *Update:* We've since moved to a property with a private well, and the difference in quality and taste is incredible—it feels more alive, more connected to the Earth.

One important tip: avoid drinking large amounts of water immediately before, during, or after meals. Doing so can dilute your stomach acid, impair digestion, and contribute to bloating, gas, or that heavy, uncomfortable feeling after eating. If you experience frequent digestive symptoms like burping, indigestion, or food sitting in your stomach too long, try taking 1–2 tablespoons of apple cider vinegar diluted in water about 20 minutes before meals. This helps support healthy stomach acid levels, which are essential for breaking down proteins and absorbing nutrients properly.

However, for those with histamine sensitivity or intolerance, apple cider vinegar may not be ideal. In that case, consider looking into Betaine HCl with pepsin as a gentle and effective alternative. Low stomach acid is far more common than people realize, and correcting it can significantly improve digestion, energy, and nutrient absorption. Do your research—this isn't a minor point. In fact, for many, supplementing with Betaine HCl has been a game-changer.

Most people (even many of the experts I've studied) don't talk about this enough: a large number of stomach acid issues, including GERD and acid reflux, actually stem from a dysregulated vagus nerve and low vagal tone. When someone experiences chronic stress, PTSD, burnout, or insomnia, the nervous system becomes unbalanced, and the vagus nerve can't function properly. One of its jobs is to regulate the esophageal sphincter—the valve that's supposed to stay closed to keep stomach acid from rising. When vagal tone is low, that sphincter may relax at the wrong times, allowing acid to move upward and cause discomfort. So, while we often hear that reflux is caused by "too much acid," in many cases, it's more about poor nerve regulation than excess acid.

Healing the vagus nerve and nervous system as a whole can be a powerful part of resolving these digestive issues at the root. Vitamin B1 deficiency can affect nerve and vagus nerve conduction as well. Dr. Eric Berg also has some great insights on stomach acid that I recommend checking out. For more information about Vitamin B1, I recommend research conducted by Dr. Darren Schmidt and nutritionist

Elliot Overton. If you're experiencing symptoms of leaky gut or more serious digestive imbalances, stomach acid support alone may not be enough. That's when a more comprehensive approach—going on the GAPS Diet or using targeted gut healing protocols—becomes necessary.

To continue this water element in diet, let's talk about meat broth, which is extremely important for gut health and the whole body. Meat broth is one of the most soothing, nourishing, and foundational healing foods, especially when it comes to gut health and immune support. Unlike long–cooked bone broth, meat broth is made by simmering cuts of meat that still contain bone, skin, connective tissue and fat for a shorter amount of time (typically 1.5 to 3 hours). This results in a lighter, more easily digestible broth that is rich in amino acids like glycine and proline, as well as collagen and gelatin, which help seal and repair the gut lining—critical for anyone dealing with leaky gut, chronic inflammation, or digestive discomfort.

Meat broth is also calming to the nervous system and gentle on the stomach, making it ideal for those recovering from illness or dealing with autoimmune or stress–related disorders. It's hydrating, mineral–rich and can be easily enhanced with healing ingredients like sea salt, herbs, or a splash of sauerkraut juice for added probiotics. Starting your day with warm meat broth provides your body with the nourishment and grounding it needs to begin healing from the inside out.

Mentally and emotionally, the water element expresses itself through qualities like adaptability, fluidity, and emotional flexibility. To embody the water element means being able to "go with the flow," responding to life's changes with grace rather than resistance. Just as water finds its way around obstacles, those aligned with this element can navigate emotional challenges with a sense of ease and trust. Water teaches us the art of allowing and of letting go, rather than clinging or forcing outcomes. This principle is deeply reflected in Buddhist philosophy, where concepts like non–attachment, surrender, and living in harmony with the present moment closely mirror the essence of water. It's about yielding, not because of weakness, but because of wisdom.

Water also symbolizes connection. In our bodies, water binds and supports every system from circulation to detoxification to communication between cells. In the world around us, water connects ecosystems across the surface of the earth, beneath it, and even in the sky through rain and vapor. Similarly, our emotional lives are nourished by connection to community, to loved ones, and to the rhythms of nature. A well-balanced water element supports deep emotional intelligence, compassion, and the ability to form strong, supportive relationships. When water is in harmony within us, we feel more connected, intuitive, and capable of embracing life's flow with trust and emotional resilience. Please try to always intend to have a balance between Earth and Water elements and especially between Water and Fire.

As always, listen to your body, go at your own pace, and stay curious. Hydration is more than just drinking water—it's about absorbing and circulating life force throughout your body. Water carries information, emotion, and energy. Make it pure, make it mindful.

Air – The Power of Breath, Mind, and Movement

In nature, the wind represents movement, change, and the invisible forces that shape the world around us. It carries seeds across vast distances, shifts weather patterns, and clears away stagnant energy. Without the flow of air, nature would become stagnant and lifeless. Wind brings renewal, stirs the trees, freshens the environment, and supports life in constant motion. Similarly, within the body and mind, the element of air governs breath, clarity, and mental agility.

The Power of Breath

Deep breathing is one of the most powerful and accessible tools we have for calming the nervous system, improving circulation, and enhancing overall vitality. When done with intention, breath acts like a reset switch for both the body and the mind. I recommend making it a daily habit to take several deep diaphragmatic breaths, especially when you first wake up, before meals, or right before sleep.

Breathing through the nose is especially important. Nasal breathing naturally produces nitric oxide, a molecule essential for proper blood flow, oxygen absorption, and immune function. It also helps regulate nervous system activity and pH balance. When you want to calm your body and mind, slow your breath and allow each inhale and exhale to be deep and smooth. This activates the vagus nerve and brings you into the parasympathetic "rest and digest" state, where healing, repair, and emotional regulation can occur.

If you're looking for energy during the day, try to keep breathing light and even through the nose. Over–breathing or excessive deep breathing when it's not needed can sometimes dysregulate your nervous system or increase fatigue, especially if your carbon dioxide levels drop too low. Tuning into your breath and adjusting it for what you need—calm or energy—is a subtle but powerful practice.

Another simple but overlooked tip is airflow while sleeping. Try cracking a window or using a fan to keep fresh air circulating at night. It's a small thing that can help improve your sleep quality and reduce the buildup of stagnant indoor air, which many people don't realize can affect mood and energy.

Mental and Emotional Air Qualities

On a mental and emotional level, air represents thought, clarity, perception, and communication. It's the element that governs our intellect, creativity, and the capacity to observe and process. Emotionally, a balanced air element allows us to step back and see things clearly without getting overwhelmed. It helps us detach from emotional chaos and observe our thoughts and reactions with curiosity and awareness.

Too much "air" can lead to feeling scattered, overthinking, anxiety, or spinning mental narratives that never settle. Not enough air can show up as brain fog, difficulty making decisions, or a lack of mental flexibility. Practices like mindfulness, breathwork, journaling, and stillness can help bring the air element into balance—keeping the mind alert but grounded.

Just as wind moves through nature to clear and renew, breath and thought can move through us to refresh and reorganize our internal world. Keep the air moving, but don't let it blow you off course. Let it guide you toward clarity, expression, and freedom.

Fire – Light for Energy, Vitality, and Balance

In nature, fire represents transformation, energy, illumination, and life force. It is the spark of movement, the heat that fuels growth, and the passion behind all living things. Without fire, there is no warmth, no light, no metabolism. And just as nature relies on fire to burn away the old and make room for new life, we rely on the fire element in our own bodies to energize us, light us up, and fuel our internal systems.

One of the simplest and most effective ways to nourish your internal fire is by stepping outside into the morning light. Within the first hour of waking, try to get at least 5–30 minutes of natural light exposure. No need to stare directly at the sun, just allow the ambient light to enter your eyes and skin. This simple ritual helps regulate your circadian rhythm, the body's internal clock that governs sleep, energy, metabolism, and hormonal cycles.

Morning sunlight benefits:
- Acts as a natural wakeup signal, boosting alertness
- Increases serotonin for improved mood and reduced anxiety
- Regulates melatonin for better sleep at night
- Enhances metabolism and immune function
- Supports natural vitamin D production

Fire in its literal form (campfires, candles, infrared light) can also provide healing benefits. Sitting near a fire is not just relaxing; the near–infrared and infrared wavelengths emitted from flames actually penetrate the skin, stimulating cellular repair and calming the nervous system. It's no coincidence that humans have gathered around fire for thousands of years; it's encoded in our biology.

Red light and Near–infrared Therapy

Red and near–infrared light therapy is one of the most valuable modern tools for physical, mental, and emotional healing. These wavelengths penetrate deeply into tissue, activating mitochondria (your body's energy centers) to produce ATP, which fuels cellular repair and detoxification. This therapy can help:

- Improve blood circulation and lymphatic drainage
- Calm the nervous system and reduce cortisol
- Support hormone regulation
- Improve sleep quality and mood
- Reduce physical tension and inflammation
- Detoxify the body by stimulating deeper tissue layers

Many people dealing with PTSD, chronic stress, or anxiety feel a significant sense of "relief" or lightness after red light sessions. It's not just placebo—your cells are literally being recharged. Used consistently and in combination with breathwork, grounding, and proper nutrition, this kind of therapy can be a powerful adjunct to your healing process.

The Fire Within – Movement, Passion, and Purpose

Fire also rules over passion, willpower, inspiration and transformation. It gives us the drive to take action, to change, to show up. Emotionally, fire shows up as determination, courage, and sometimes even anger, which, when expressed healthily, can be a sign that our boundaries need defending. But too much fire, like chronic anger, irritability, or burnout, can burn us out. Not enough, and we lack energy, motivation, and warmth.

To balance the fire element within, I practice a few simple yoga and mobility techniques every day. I don't remember that last time I went a day without some form of movement and learning. These postures are not extreme or advanced, they're grounding, energizing, and deeply restorative. They help me stay connected to my breath, my body, and my purpose. I'll walk you through some of these daily habits in the next section.

Fire reminds us to be lit up but not consumed, to stay passionate but not burned out, and to move with purpose but also with intention.

Ether – Ethereal – Spirit

Some people associate the Ether element with nature, and I do as well, but I also like to make a distinction between the natural world and the more subtle, ethereal realms: the spiritual, energetic, and unseen forces that many call Higher Power, Source, God, or even "The Heavens." In various cultures, especially in Asia and within Christian traditions, this idea is often referred to as "Heaven" or "the Heavens." When Yoda teaches Luke Skywalker about the Force, this is what he means; it's the energy that surrounds and binds all living things. This concept closely mirrors what some traditions and philosophies describe as the Ether or Spirit element.

Now, to clarify a subtle but important distinction: the element of Ether is often described as stillness, spaciousness, meditation, contemplation, reflection and the presence of the void—sometimes even the "unknown." It's not necessarily about a deity or divine being, but about the experience of pure silence, empty space, and the backdrop behind all existence. Meditation, solitude, and deep presence in nature connect us to this energy. Too much Ether, though, can sometimes bring a sense of eeriness or disconnection—like floating with no ground beneath you.

On the other hand, the concept of Spirit, God, or a Higher Power relates more to the personal and relational aspect of the divine. This is less about emptiness and more about connection, meaning purpose and the sacred. If this starts to sound a bit too abstract, just stick with the elemental understanding of Ether: stillness, spaciousness, and serenity.

Mentally and emotionally, the Ether element represents peace, calm, and presence. It's the energy of spaciousness in your mind and heart—the ability to pause, to reflect, and to simply be. Again, you don't want to become too deep into Ether because you'll be too abstract, dissociated and numb.

Whether you're sitting in quiet meditation or lying under a night sky, Ether invites you to return to the awareness that there's something bigger than your current thoughts, emotions, or struggles. It's a subtle but powerful presence, and it's always available when we make space to feel it.

Compassion, along with deep understanding, is one of the deepest expressions of the Ether element. It's not just an emotion, it's a state of being that arises from connecting to something greater than ourselves. When you tap into Ether or Spirit, you begin to feel the shared experience of being human—the joy, pain, struggle, and growth. From that space, true compassion is born. It's not forced or superficial, it's a natural response that comes when we sit in stillness and recognize that every living being is on their own journey. Compassion bridges the gap between the self and others. It softens judgment, opens the heart, and brings a quiet strength that says, "I see you." In that way, compassion becomes an energetic force—an invisible thread that connects us all.

It's worth mentioning a few more things. Sensitivity, gentleness, consciousness and that divine spark within you all fall into this category as well. These are the subtle energies that often get overlooked in a world obsessed with speed and strength, but they are powerful forces in their own right. Sensitivity isn't weakness—it's awareness. Gentleness isn't passivity—it's presence. And that divine spark? It's the part of you that remembers who you truly are beyond all the noise.

These qualities are deeply connected to Ether—the stillness behind the breath, the quiet between thoughts, the space where healing and higher guidance flow. Nurturing this part of yourself isn't about escaping reality; it's about learning to walk through it with grace, intuition, and inner alignment.

Synergy and Balance of the Elements

Let's take a moment to talk about the importance of bringing all the elements together. Each element—Earth, Water, Fire, Air, and Ether—carries its own unique energy, lessons, and healing properties. When one becomes too dominant or another is neglected, it can throw your physical, emotional, and mental health out of balance. Earth without flow can become rigid. Water without structure can become destructive. Fire without grounding and water can be chaotic and burn out or burn others. Air without direction can scatter energy. Ether without anchoring can feel disconnected or overwhelming.

True wellness and personal power come from knowing how to balance these energies within yourself. You might find that during certain seasons of life, you need more of one than another—and that's okay. The goal isn't to live in perfect harmony every second, but to continually check in, adjust, and cultivate awareness of what you're needing in the moment. Integrating the elements into your lifestyle through breath, movement, mindfulness, nutrition, and connection can bring clarity, resilience, and a deeper sense of inner peace. When the elements are in balance, you feel more like yourself. Grounded, clear, energized, compassionate, and connected.

Let's move onto some Asana – Physical posture and important poses.

SQUAT. Period. Done. Next.

That's how important squatting is for your body. It's one of the most powerful yet underused movements we have. Squatting is an ancient posture and natural position that supports nearly every system in your body. Squats are phenomenal hip openers and support the groin, legs, calves, ankles, spine, lymphatic system, core, and even your breath. It's not just an exercise, it's a foundation.

I squat first thing in the morning. I'll squat when I go outside for morning sunlight. I'll squat randomly during the day, especially when I feel tightness in my hips, back, or legs. It helps relieve lower back pain and stiffness. And here's the key: aim to squat with your feet flat on the ground. If you can't yet, that's okay. Just keep at it every day, and your mobility will improve with time.

Sometimes I just hold a deep squat and take a few breaths to engage my diaphragm and those deeper intercostal breathing muscles. Other times, I'll do a quick set of squats—try five partial reps, halfway down. If you can only do one full squat, that's your starting point. Build from there. I've had to start from zero more than once. I used to be an athlete with an over 5–foot high flying sidekick. But anxiety and panic took me out. I've been flattened and I know what it's like to have to rebuild. If you're there now, I see you.

Deep Diaphragmatic Breathing

We've talked about this already, and it's worth repeating: if you want to regulate your nervous system and feel balanced, you *must* work with your breath. Especially in the evenings, or during quiet breaks, take time to practice slow, intentional belly breathing. It anchors you in the present moment and signals safety to your nervous system.

Inversions: Get Your Heart Above Your Head

This next tool is all about perspective—literally. Inversions are any position where your heart is higher than your head. Think downward dog, legs–up–the–wall, forward folds, or more advanced poses like headstands or shoulder stands. These positions offer powerful benefits, both physically and mentally.

Inversions improve circulation by helping blood flow toward the brain and heart, increasing oxygen delivery and encouraging lymphatic drainage—your body's internal detox system. They also support immune function and can relieve tension and swelling in the lower body.

But the benefits don't stop there. Inversions stimulate the parasympathetic nervous system—your rest-and-digest state—and activate the vagus nerve, which helps calm the mind and reduce cortisol levels. You'll feel more relaxed, more present, and mentally clearer. Inversions also stimulate the endocrine system, including the thyroid and adrenal glands, which help regulate energy, metabolism, and mood.

From a structural standpoint, they can decompress the spine and alleviate pressure from sitting all day. Hanging in gentle inversions can create space between the vertebrae, improving posture and reducing back pain. And let's not forget the mental aspect—being upside down can improve concentration, coordination, and inner confidence. It takes focus and trust, which builds resilience over time.

If you're new to this, start slow. Use props, walls, or try simple versions like putting your legs up on a chair or wall. Even the smallest inversion has big effects. And when practiced mindfully, inversions can become one of your most reliable tools for physical and emotional reset.

Important Yoga Poses for Daily Practice

Lunges are excellent for building lower body strength, targeting the quadriceps, hamstrings, and glutes while also enhancing balance and stability. They engage the core and improve hip mobility, which is essential for proper posture and injury prevention. Additionally, lunges help activate the hip flexors, which often become tight due to prolonged sitting, making them an important movement for counteracting sedentary lifestyles. Regularly incorporating lunges can also improve functional movement patterns, making everyday activities like walking, climbing stairs, and lifting objects easier and more efficient.

Downward facing dog is a powerful full–body stretch that lengthens the spine, opens the shoulders, and strengthens the arms, legs, and core. This pose promotes better circulation by encouraging blood flow toward the brain, which can help improve focus and reduce stress. It also stretches the hamstrings and calves while relieving tension in the lower back. By engaging the hands and feet evenly, downward dog encourages proper weight distribution and alignment, reducing strain on the wrists and lower body while enhancing overall flexibility. Holding this position also allows the nervous system to calm down, making it a great pose for relaxation and stress relief.

Spinal twists are highly effective for improving spinal mobility and releasing tension in the back. These movements help to realign the spine, reduce stiffness, and promote better posture. By gently compressing and then releasing different areas of the torso, twists stimulate digestion and support detoxification by aiding the natural movement of fluids in the organs. They also help relieve discomfort from prolonged sitting by counteracting the effects of spinal compression and improving overall range of motion. Twisting movements engage the core muscles and encourage deeper breathing, further supporting relaxation and overall spinal health. Try this every night before bed along with some deep breathing.

To recap, I chose these six yoga techniques for you to start doing everyday. You decide how much you can do. These can easily be done in between any other activities, in the morning and at night time.

IMPORTANT NOTE:
When performing yoga postures, apply what you've learned so far. This is why attending yoga classes or following guided sequences online can be beneficial. Teachers will remind you to breathe and stay present in each posture. Over time, this practice helps train both the body and mind to recognize that you are safe,

allowing you to cultivate a sense of calm and inner peace. However, if you experience any pain at any point, stop immediately. Try adjusting the posture, explore a modified version, or move on to a different technique. If needed, take a break entirely until you feel ready to continue. yoga is not about pushing through pain—it is not a "no pain, no gain" practice.

Yoga is also a mindfulness practice, encouraging deeper introspection. However, not many experts acknowledge that this can be overwhelming for those dealing with anxiety or PTSD. I personally had to approach my practice slowly, and at times, I pushed myself too hard. While mindfulness and intentional movement are valuable, sometimes it's just as beneficial to simply practice without overthinking. Some days, you may want to focus on being fully present, moving with awareness and purpose. Other days, it might be best to let go of expectations and just move through the physical techniques without analyzing them. Let the postures work their magic without overcomplicating the process. Finding this balance is an important part of the journey.

More Benefits of Yoga and Stretching

Stretching the muscles through yoga, paired with deep breathing and focused awareness, is a powerful combination for easing PTSD, stress, and anxiety. When the body stretches mindfully, it signals the nervous system that it's safe to relax. This gentle release of physical tension mirrors the release of emotional tension, helping to unwind stored stress held in the muscles, fascia, and even internal organs. For those with PTSD or chronic anxiety, where the body often remains stuck in a state of fight–or–flight, these movements help shift the system toward rest, healing, and recovery.

Deep breathing during yoga enhances this effect by activating the parasympathetic nervous system, which lowers heart rate, reduces cortisol levels, and brings the body into a more calm and grounded state. Focused, slow movements bring your attention back into the body—this somatic awareness is especially important for trauma healing, as it helps rebuild the connection between mind and body, that connection which trauma often disrupts.

> **IMPORTAT NOTE:**
> Sometimes stretching or physical activity can begin to release stored emotions and energy held in the body. When this happens, it may bring unresolved feelings to the surface, which can be triggering or uncomfortable. If this occurs, take it as a sign that your body is processing— this is part of healing. But if it feels like too much, take baby steps. Gently remind yourself that you are safe in this moment and try to breathe through it. If it becomes overwhelming, it's absolutely okay to pause and come back to it later. Often, when you return, the intensity of the trigger has already softened or may no longer be present at all. Be patient with yourself. This is a process, not a race.

Yoga–based stretching also improves circulation, joint mobility, and energy flow, supporting both physical and emotional resilience. Over time, this practice helps individuals feel more in control of their body, more emotionally stable, and better equipped to respond to stress in a calm, centered way. It's not just exercise; it's a moving therapy that can gently reset the whole system.

Other Notable Yoga Poses

Child's Pose (Balasana) is a deeply calming and restful posture that encourages the body to relax and the mind to turn inward. By gently folding forward and resting the forehead on the ground, it releases tension from the back, shoulders, and nervous system, offering a sense of safety and rest. This is ideal for easing anxiety and emotional overwhelm.

Legs–Up–the–Wall (Viparita Karani) is a gentle inversion where you lie on your back with your sacrum (tailbone, buttock area) as close to the wall as possible so that you can rest both legs vertically against a wall. This posture encourages circulation, calms the lower body, and helps reset the nervous system. It's especially helpful for reducing anxiety, fatigue, and nervous tension.

Cat–Cow Pose (Marjaryasana/Bitilasana) involves a slow flow between arching and rounding the spine while syncing movement with breath. This dynamic posture relieves spinal tension and brings awareness to the body and breath, helping calm racing thoughts and emotional restlessness.

Seated Forward Fold (Paschimottanasana) is a grounding posture that stretches the spine and back of the legs while encouraging a state of quiet introspection. It helps soothe the nervous system, slow the heart rate, and release emotional heaviness—perfect for winding down.

Supine Twist (Supta Matsyendrasana) is performed while lying on the back with the knees gently dropped to one side. This pose releases tightness in the spine and hips, supports digestion, and helps clear stagnant emotional energy, creating a sense of ease and spaciousness.

Bridge Pose (Setu Bandhasana) is a heart–opening posture that strengthens the legs and glutes while gently lifting the chest. It helps stimulate the calming parasympathetic nervous system, improves mood, and supports emotional balance by opening areas where stress is often held.

Standing Forward Fold (Uttanasana) is a powerful yet simple pose that allows the body to hang forward, encouraging a gentle release through the spine, neck, and shoulders. This posture promotes a sense of grounding, supports nervous system regulation, and brings fresh blood flow to the brain—helping to ease mental fatigue and emotional pressure.

Be sure to keep a soft bend in the knees to protect the lower back and hamstrings, especially if you're just beginning. From here, you can transition into a flat–back position (also called Ardha Uttanasana) by keeping your legs in place and bringing your spine parallel to the ground. Extend the crown of your head forward, keep your neck long, and gaze softly downward. Take a couple of deep breaths here to lengthen the spine, then gently exhale and release back down into the full forward fold.

This simple combination of alternating between the forward fold and flat back helps decompress the spine, calm the mind, and connect breath to movement. A great daily reset for body and mind.

Corpse Pose (Savasana) is the final resting posture of most yoga sessions, where you lie flat on your back in complete stillness. Though simple, it's deeply restorative and allows the nervous system to reset and the body to fully absorb the calming effects of the practice.

Practicing these poses regularly, even just for a few minutes each day, can significantly help reduce anxiety, ease symptoms of stress, and support emotional wellbeing. When combined with deep breathing and mindful awareness, they become powerful tools for healing and inner peace.

Bedtime and Sleep Routine

It's good for everyone to have a healthy bedtime routine. Creating a healthy bedtime routine is one of the most powerful ways to improve your sleep, regulate your nervous system, and support overall mental and physical health. In a world filled with overstimulation from screens, stress, noise, and constant activity, your body and mind need a clear signal that it's time to wind down. A consistent nightly routine helps transition you out of the alert, high–stress state (sympathetic mode) and into the rest–and–repair state (parasympathetic mode), which is essential for deep, restorative sleep. Let's go through some basics that you can customize to what works best for you.

One of the most effective tools for this transition is incorporating gentle yoga and breathing into your bedtime routine. Yoga for sleep isn't about working up a sweat or challenging your flexibility. It's about slowing down, grounding your energy, and preparing the body and mind for rest. Gentle stretches like legs–up–the–wall, child's pose, seated forward fold, and spinal twists help release tension stored in the hips, lower back, shoulders, and nervous system. These movements signal safety to the brain, calm the heart rate, and improve circulation—all of which are vital for high–quality sleep.

Pairing these movements with slow, deep breathing, especially belly breathing or extended exhalations, helps activate the vagus nerve, which tells the body it's time to relax. You might lie down in a supported position like reclined butterfly or savasana, place one hand on your belly and one on your chest and focus on breathing slowly through the nose for several minutes. Adding in a short meditation or body scan can further deepen the calming effect.

A few other helpful elements to add to your nighttime ritual include turning off screens at least an hour before bed, dimming the lights to signal melatonin production, drinking a warm non–caffeinated herbal tea, writing in a gratitude journal, or reading something light and peaceful. Try to go to bed around the same time each night and allow yourself at least 30–60 minutes of "slow down" time before actually getting into bed.

This bedtime practice is more than just preparing for sleep. It tells your body and mind, "You are safe now." It's okay to rest." In the context of PTSD, anxiety, or chronic illness, this kind of nightly self–care can be a healing anchor, helping retrain the brain and body to feel calm, grounded, and capable of deep, healing sleep. This may sound a bit quirky but the more you tell your body it's time to sleep and relax, the more it will listen to you. You may or may not want to do a journal entry late at night, so think about whether this will help you or maybe it's best to do something like that during the daytime. Or if something comes up and journaling helps, then go ahead but just feel it out for yourself.

Taking care of yourself before bed: bring some loving attention to your sweet, beautiful feet. Spend a few minutes gently massaging your soles, the inner arches, each toe, and between the toes. Work up to the top of the feet, gliding between the tendons, and don't forget the outer edges. Finish by circling up around the inner ankle bone and along the soft inner ankle, then trace upward along the inside of the shinbone. It's grounding, calming, and just feels nice.

I usually follow this with a soothing belly massage—light to moderate pressure in slow, clockwise circles around the navel. The goal is to release the fascia (the connective tissue beneath the skin), which can hold onto stress like emotional velcro. The more you do this, the more you'll dial in the pressure and rhythm that works for you. You'll be surprised how much tension is stored in the gut. If you're still feeling up for it, end with a gentle massage at the back of the neck and just under the base of the skull. This little ritual can help settle your nervous system and guide you into deeper, more restful sleep. A proper ending to your day is a little healing and a whole lot of self–care.

Chakras (The Body's Energy Centers)

If the idea of chakras feels a little too much like *woo–woo* for you, just hang with me for a moment before you skip this section. My motto is simple: if it works, use it.

Some people are just more energy sensitive than others. There's absolutely zero judgment here—whether you can or can't feel or sense energy doesn't make you better or worse than anyone else. If this topic sparks your curiosity, there are plenty of directions you can explore beyond this book, including countless books on the subject and searching for a good teacher. Personally, I first learned about chakras through Qigong, yoga, Reiki, Shamanic work, and various books and teachers over the years. I've done healing work both for others and for myself, and I can tell you, when used well, this approach can be incredibly helpful. I've used it both for putting out fires in the moment and for helping to heal deeper, root-level issues.

One quick note: please don't get overly caught up in the whole "energy" thing or feel like you need to master it. It's just one tool, nothing more, nothing less. Some people naturally tune into this kind of work; others don't. That's okay. We're all wired differently, different personalities, different bodies, different constitutions. You get the picture. Take what works or makes sense for you and leave the rest.

7 Main Chakras

Root Chakra (Muladhara)
Located: Base of the spine
Theme: Safety, survival, grounding

When someone is dealing with PTSD or anxiety, the root chakra is often out of balance. It's tied to your basic sense of safety and feeling connected to the earth and your body. If you're always in fight-or-flight, your nervous system literally doesn't feel safe here. Symptoms of imbalance might include hypervigilance, restlessness, fear of instability (housing, finances, relationships), or even physical tension in the legs, hips, and lower back. Practices like grounding, breathwork, and reconnecting to the physical body can help restore balance.

Sacral Chakra (Svadhisthana)
Located: Lower abdomen, about two inches below the navel
Theme: Emotions, pleasure, creativity

PTSD and trauma often lock the body in survival mode, shutting down this chakra's flow. It governs healthy emotional expression and the ability to experience pleasure. Many trauma survivors struggle here, feeling emotionally numb or emotionally overwhelmed, with blocked creativity or sexual energy. Releasing tension in the hips and pelvis, practicing joyful movement, or creative expression can begin to help restore this flow.

Solar Plexus Chakra (Manipura)
Located: Upper abdomen/stomach area
Theme: Personal power, willpower, self-worth

This chakra often takes a hit when living with chronic stress or trauma. The solar plexus is tied to your sense of personal power, your ability to act, assert boundaries, and feel in control of your life. With PTSD or anxiety, it's common to feel powerless or stuck in cycles of self-doubt. Physically, it can show up as digestive issues or a "knot" in the stomach. Building confidence, taking small actions, and strengthening boundaries help restore balance here.

Heart Chakra (Anahata)
Located: Center of the chest
Theme: Love, compassion, connection

Trauma often leads to guardedness or emotional withdrawal, which constricts the heart chakra. It governs your ability to give and receive love—not just romantically, but connection with others and yourself. Many people with PTSD feel disconnected or numb here. Practices that promote self-compassion, forgiveness, and safe, authentic relationships help reopen this center. Breathwork aimed at the heart space can also support healing.

Throat Chakra (Vishuddha)
Located: Throat
Theme: Communication, self-expression, truth

When trauma affects the throat chakra, it can manifest as difficulty speaking one's truth, fear of being heard, or trouble expressing emotions. Many survivors learned to stay silent to stay safe. This can show up physically as tightness in the throat, jaw tension, or voice issues. Gently reclaiming your voice—through speaking, writing, singing, or simply giving yourself permission to say "no" or "yes"—helps restore this energy center.

Third Eye Chakra (Ajna)
Located: Forehead, between the eyebrows
Theme: Intuition, insight, mental clarity

PTSD and anxiety can create a mind that's in constant overdrive, hypervigilant, racing, or stuck in fear-based patterns. This disrupts the third eye chakra, which governs clarity, intuition, and perspective. When this chakra is imbalanced, people often feel lost in fear or disconnected from their inner wisdom. Meditation, mindfulness, and calming breathwork can help bring this center back into balance, allowing clearer thinking and greater inner trust.

Crown Chakra (Sahasrara)
Located: Top of the head
Theme: Connection to higher purpose, meaning, and inner peace

Trauma can leave people feeling disconnected from life, spirit, and meaning. The crown chakra is about the bigger picture—feeling connected to something beyond yourself. For some, that may be spiritual or religious; for others, it's about purpose or contribution. When this chakra is blocked, people often feel hopeless or spiritually disconnected. Mindful practices, nature, gratitude, and even simple acts of kindness can help reopen this pathway toward a deeper sense of connection and peace.

The main chakras I've worked with—and still do from time to time—are the root, solar plexus, and heart chakras. One simple thing you can try is placing your hands over the chakra you're focusing on, with the intention to cleanse, heal, balance, and strengthen that energy center. You don't have to overthink it, just bring positive thoughts and a gentle focus to that area. You can also adjust your intention slightly depending on the chakra. For example, you might focus on stability with the root chakra, personal power with the solar plexus, or self-compassion with the heart. Even just reflecting on what we covered earlier about each chakra can help bring awareness, insight, and healing to those areas.

The chakras and Dan Tians in Qigong can also be worked with in connection, supporting each other as part of your overall energy system. You'll learn more about that in the next chapter.

Takeaways from Chapter 8:

- Yoga is an ancient practice that has been proven over thousands of years to support the mind, body and spirit in many ways.
- Yoga doesn't have to be done 90 minutes a day or even an hour a day to receive benefits. You can start small or build it into your lifestyle as you see fit. Sometimes, even just a few minutes several times a day, or 15 minutes a day can be very beneficial. Something, anything is better than nothing!
- Start building little strategies for a healthier lifestyle with the elements like earth, fire, air, water, and ethereal. You can do all of them within 5 minutes of waking up.
- Start doing a handful of the daily techniques and build from there. Make a list and run through it every day, even doing a few will create change.
- Yoga was originally a part of everyone's daily routine, exercise and martial arts practice. It just got separated over the years.
- Chakra work can be a great tool for your "toolbox."
- Finish your happy day with a nice self-care routine.

Chapter 9
QiGong – Embodiment and Feeling Safe

"When I let go of what I am, I become what I might be."
— *Lao Tzu*

Qigong, an ancient Chinese practice, combines movement, meditation, and controlled breathing to cultivate and balance the body's vital energy, known as "qi" or "chi." Rooted in traditional Chinese medicine, philosophy, and martial arts, Qigong is designed to promote physical and mental health, improve flexibility, and enhance overall wellbeing. The practice involves a series of postures, gentle exercises, and meditative breathing techniques that can be tailored to individual needs and abilities.

Qigong is often referred to as the "art of effortless power," highlighting its focus on natural, flowing movements that enhance the body's energy flow without causing strain. This practice not only improves physical strength and flexibility but also fosters mental clarity and emotional stability. Through regular practice, Qigong helps in reducing stress, boosting the immune system, and increasing vitality.

Understanding Yin and Yang: The Balance of Life

Yin and Yang are the two fundamental energies that make up everything in the universe. These forces originate from the "void," the infinite stillness or potential from which all things arise. Together, Yin and Yang represent balance, polarity, and interdependence. Yin is often associated with the feminine and the cool, dark, passive, and receptive qualities of existence. Yang, on the other hand, embodies the masculine, and the warm, bright, active, and expressive aspects of life.

When these energies are in balance, there is harmony in the body, mind, and world around us. However, when one dominates the other, imbalance and disharmony begin to manifest. For example, too much Yin without enough Yang to balance it can lead to excessive passivity, overthinking, emotional heaviness, fatigue, and physical stagnation. In practical terms, it might look like constantly staying still, getting lost in emotions without taking action, or falling into patterns of withdrawal and inaction.

For the modern world (and yes, for all the gamers sitting in dark basements), this could mean spending too much time in stillness or comfort zones, lacking movement, ambition, or motivation to take on life's challenges. From the perspective of Chinese medicine, this would be seen as Qi stagnation, not enough energetic movement or blood flow in the body, leading to issues like low energy, poor digestion, chronic fatigue, or even depression.

While Yin qualities like introspection, rest, and emotional depth are essential, they must be balanced with Yang qualities like initiative, movement, and assertiveness. Life requires both rest and action, stillness and motion, feeling and doing. Yang energy drives us to get up, move forward, create, build, and transform. It is the energy that pushes life forward, that meets challenges with courage, that steps into the unknown.

To live in harmony with the Yin–Yang dynamic is to understand when to rest and when to act, when to feel and when to do, when to reflect and when to take charge. This balance is not fixed; it's fluid and ever–changing. The wisdom lies in learning to listen to your body, your energy, and the rhythm of your life, and knowing when it's time to flow and when it's time to rise.

The Five Aspects of Qigong: A Path to Inner Harmony

Qigong is more than just a set of slow movements, it is a holistic practice designed to harmonize the body, energy, and consciousness. One of its foundational principles is the progression through five aspects of calming: calm the body, calm the breath, calm the energy, calm the mind, and calm the spirit. These layers are deeply interconnected, each one building upon the next to create a state of inner balance, health, and presence.

Calm the body is the first and most tangible step. By releasing physical tension, improving posture, and moving with intention, the body becomes a stable and relaxed foundation. Without a calm body, the nervous system remains on high alert, making it difficult to access deeper states of awareness or healing.

From there, we move into calm the breath. The breath acts as a bridge between the body and the mind. When breath becomes slow, smooth, and natural, it sends a signal to the brain that it is safe to relax. In Qigong, the breath becomes a tool to regulate emotions, enhance energy flow, and ground awareness in the present moment.

Once the breath is calm, we begin to calm the energy (Qi). This is when the internal flow of life force becomes more organized and smooth. The practitioner begins to feel the subtle currents of Qi moving through the body, unblocking stagnation and nourishing the organs and tissues. Calm energy feels expansive, light, and vibrant.

This leads naturally into calming the mind. As the body, breath, and energy settle, the mind also begins to quiet. Mental chatter slows down, and the practitioner experiences greater clarity, focus, and emotional steadiness. A calm mind is not empty, but peaceful and aware, free from the grip of distraction or stress.

Finally, we reach calm the spirit, a deep sense of stillness, connection, and presence. This is not something that can be forced, but something that arises when all other aspects are in harmony. The spirit, or *Shen*, reflects our higher awareness, our sense of purpose, and our inner light. When the spirit is calm, we feel aligned with ourselves and with life itself.

Together, these five aspects form a powerful system of self-regulation, healing, and awakening. Practicing Qigong with this framework allows the practitioner to move from the outer world to the inner, from the physical to the spiritual, creating a deep and lasting sense of harmony.

Once the spirit is calm and flowing, a person becomes both inspired and inspiring. Their eyes glisten with clarity and presence. They feel deeply motivated and naturally uplift those around them. There is a sense of purpose that runs through them—not just as an idea, but as a lived experience. In this state, they are not just existing; they are truly living their purpose.

Three Principles of QiGong

In Qigong, the principles of purge, tonify, and regulate form a core framework for restoring and maintaining energetic balance in the body. These three steps work together to help clear stagnation, build strength, and harmonize the flow of Qi (life force energy) throughout the body's meridians and organ systems. This can be applied in generally any area of life.

Purging is the first step, and it involves releasing what no longer serves the body or mind such as stagnant energy, emotional tension, pain, toxins, and even excess heat or dampness in traditional Chinese medicine terms. Movements that shake, twist, stretch, or exhale with force are often used to clear blockages and open the body's channels, creating space for new energy to flow. This stage is especially helpful for people dealing with stress, anger, grief, or chronic tension.

Once the body is cleared, the second step is to tonify, or nourish. This means building and replenishing vital energy in areas that are depleted, whether that's the organs, blood, immune system, or overall vitality. Gentle flowing movements, breathwork, and visualization are used to draw in fresh Qi from nature or the universe, filling the body's reservoirs and strengthening its core. This is where healing and rejuvenation begin to take place.

The final step is to regulate, bringing the body, mind, and energy systems into balance. This stage harmonizes the opposing forces of Yin and Yang, balances excess or deficiency, and helps maintain smooth, steady energy flow. Regulation is what allows the effects of purging and tonifying to integrate fully, so that the benefits can be sustained long-term.

Together, purging, tonifying, and regulating create a full-spectrum approach to energetic health, clearing out what's harmful, building up what's needed, and ensuring everything flows in harmony.

Here are a few practical examples of how the principles of purge, tonify, and regulate can be used in real life, especially for someone dealing with PTSD, anxiety, or chronic stress:

Purge – Releasing Emotional or Physical Tension

For someone with anxiety or PTSD, tension can build up in the body and nervous system, often without even realizing it. You might carry tightness in your shoulders, clench your jaw, or feel heavy in your chest. A simple purging practice could be shaking the body gently, twisting the spine, or using forceful exhalations (like a "ha" breath) while swinging the arms. These movements help to discharge nervous energy, release trapped emotions and reduce the feeling of being "stuck" in a heightened state of stress or fear. You can find these types of QiGong exercises online by easily typing these keywords in like (gentle Qigong purging techniques).

One of the biggest philosophies in Buddhism is "letting go." So simply practice mentally letting things go that don't serve you anymore, even though that sounds cliché, it's a very strong technique that's survived thousands of years at this point.

Tonify – Rebuilding After Exhaustion

People with PTSD and chronic anxiety often feel drained or fatigued after intense emotional periods or hypervigilance. Tonifying practices involve slow, nourishing Qigong movements, deep abdominal breathing, and visualizing energy flowing in from nature or the Earth into the body. A great example is standing in Wuji posture while imagining golden light filling the lower belly (Lower Dan Tian), slowly building your inner energy. This helps restore vitality, boost the immune system, and rebuild a sense of inner safety and strength. Also think about eating a more robust diet, like what you read about earlier in the chapter about different diets with strong bioavailable vitamins and minerals. Think about increasing your friend circle or having stronger bonds with others.

Regulate – Creating Balance and Stability

After releasing and replenishing energy, it's essential to regulate the system so the changes can integrate. This helps bring emotional steadiness and physical harmony. A regulating practice might be mindful breathing with gentle movement, such as spinal waves or slow, circular arm movements, done with smooth breath and focused awareness. This stage is key for someone with PTSD, as it teaches the nervous system how to settle into a new, calmer baseline, rather than swinging between extremes of hyperarousal and shutdown.

By regularly practicing this cycle—purging what weighs you down, tonifying what lifts you up, and regulating to maintain the balance—you're giving your body and mind the tools to heal, stabilize, and become more resilient. It's a gentle yet powerful system for working with trauma and stress in a grounded, embodied way.

The last thing I want to share here is the Qigong technique of **"forgetting."** This refers to the practice of letting go, mentally, emotionally, and physically. You don't literally forget, but it's about releasing the need to control, overthink, or cling to outcomes. In practice, it means entering a movement or meditation without forcing, analyzing, or trying too hard, simply allowing the body to move and the breath to flow while the mind gently releases its grip. This creates space for natural healing, presence, and inner stillness. For those with anxiety, PTSD, or stress, "forgetting" helps interrupt mental loops and invites a return to the body, the breath, and the now. It's not about avoiding, but about allowing things to settle by not holding on so tightly.

Qigong and the Importance of Physical Posture: Aligning the 18 Parts of the Body.

One of the most essential yet often overlooked aspects of Qigong is posture. Proper alignment isn't just about looking graceful; it's about creating an open and relaxed structure through which Qi (energy) can flow freely.

The body in Qigong is understood as a system of interconnected parts, often broken down into 18 key alignment points. When each part is correctly positioned, the body becomes stable, open, and energy-efficient, reducing strain, enhancing circulation, and allowing the practitioner to cultivate energy with ease. Misalignment in even one area can block the flow of Qi and lead to physical discomfort or energetic stagnation.

Here's a breakdown of the 18 essential parts of the body in Qigong posture and how each should be aligned:

1. Top of the Head (Baihui Point) – lightly lifted upward as if a string is pulling it toward the sky. This opens the spine and connects the body to Heaven energy.
2. Forehead – relaxed, free from tension. Mental tension often collects here, so soften it.
3. Eyebrows and Eyes – eyebrows relaxed, gaze soft and unfocused, usually directed slightly downward. Eyes stay open but calm, like you're seeing but not staring.
4. Mouth – gently closed or slightly open, with the tongue resting on the roof of the mouth behind the upper teeth (creating an energy circuit).
5. Jaw – unclenched and relaxed. Tension here can radiate throughout the head and neck.
6. Neck – lengthened and aligned, not tilted forward or back. The chin should be slightly tucked to elongate the spine.

7. Shoulders – relaxed and dropped, not hunched. This opens the chest and helps relieve tension.
8. Elbows – slightly bent and soft, never locked. They should feel like they're gently floating.
9. Wrists – relaxed, with a sense of suspension. Avoid stiffness.
10. Hands/Fingers – naturally open with a slight curve, as if holding a ball. Fingers shouldn't be rigid or limp.
11. Chest – soft and open, not puffed out. This allows for deep, natural breathing and opens the heart center.
12. Upper Back – rounded slightly and relaxed. Avoid excessive arching or collapsing.
13. Lower Back – lengthened and neutral, not overly arched. A slight pelvic tuck often helps align this area.
14. Abdomen – soft and relaxed. The breath should naturally move here, expanding the belly without force.
15. Pelvis – neutral and aligned, like a bowl holding water—neither tilted forward nor backward.
16. Hips – relaxed and slightly sunk, grounding the body. Tension here restricts flow to the lower body.
17. Knees – slightly bent, never locked. This keeps energy flowing and connects upper and lower body.
18. Feet – flat on the ground, hip–width apart (or shoulder–width depending on the form), with weight evenly distributed. The "Yongquan" point on the sole is the root—your connection to Earth energy.

Correct alignment of these 18 parts creates a posture that is both stable and relaxed, allowing for energetic flow, emotional calm, and mental clarity. Over time, practicing Qigong with mindful attention to posture not only improves physical health by reducing tension, improving circulation, and supporting joint health, but also helps harmonize the mind and spirit.

In Qigong, posture is more than just structure, it's the vessel through which life energy flows, connecting Heaven and Earth through the body. By aligning yourself daily, you tune your system like a finely crafted instrument, ready to resonate with health, peace, and power.

Both nutrition and mental health are closely connected to posture, forming a powerful trio that influences overall wellbeing. Interestingly, in the Dutch language, the word for posture translates to "attitude," which beautifully reflects the deeper truth that how we carry ourselves physically often mirrors how we feel mentally and emotionally. When posture is misaligned, whether due to habit, stress, or physical imbalances, it can disrupt more than just our appearance.

Poor posture affects breathing, limiting the diaphragm's ability to expand fully, which reduces oxygen intake and can lead to fatigue, brain fog, and even heightened anxiety. Misalignment in the feet, hips, spine, shoulders, and neck can ripple up or down through the entire body, contributing to issues such as joint pain, poor digestion, and chronic tension. Over time, these physical imbalances can also influence our mood, self-esteem, and mental clarity. Not to mention, degradation of joints and tissues.

Conversely, standing or sitting with an upright, balanced posture supports better circulation, digestion, and nervous system function, while also promoting a greater sense of confidence and emotional stability. When paired with proper nutrition, which provides the essential building blocks for energy, focus, and recovery, the body becomes more resilient and the mind clearer. Caring for your posture is not just a physical habit; it's an act of self-respect and a direct path to improved mental and emotional wellbeing.

In the same way, healthy eating habits help prevent nutritional deficiencies, as discussed in Chapter 3. Consuming collagen-rich foods and following an animal-based diet can supply the body with the nutrients necessary for maintaining healthy joints, muscles, tissues, and skin. This type of nourishment also plays a key role in reducing inflammation, supporting overall vitality and reinforcing the body's natural healing processes.

I advise you to watch some YouTube videos on this, there are so many out there. Also, you can have someone stand next you and tell you if you are standing straight or not. Or get video of yourself. Many people stand forward leaning and don't know it. A little is okay, but chronic misalignment is where trouble lies.

Golden Ball

This here is a very basic explanation and understanding of the Golden Ball exercise. This gets into an area of energetics. Some of this might not make sense to you, but for some it might make perfect sense. Some people are "energy sensitive" while others "don't feel a thing." Either way, it's okay! If this isn't for you, just simply move along to the next chapter or the next thing that resonates with you. Again, this is part of my healing process and I'm sharing what helped me in hopes that it might help you. Some of the "energetic" stuff often needs to be experienced before learning about it, so let's dive into the basics!

The Golden Ball exercise is a foundational and deeply nourishing practice in Qigong, designed to cultivate, gather, and circulate life force energy (the Qi) throughout the body. At first glance, it may seem simple: the practitioner stands still, holding their arms in a rounded position as if cradling a large, glowing ball of energy between the hands. But beneath its stillness lies profound power. This exercise helps to activate the body's energy centers, align posture, calm the mind, and strengthen the flow of Qi through the meridians.

In this posture, the arms form a gentle arc, usually held at chest level (or sometimes at the lower abdomen), with the fingers relaxed and slightly spread as if holding an actual ball of light. The knees are soft, the spine is upright, the shoulders are relaxed, and the breath is natural and deep, flowing into the belly. The Golden Ball is both a standing meditation and an energy–building technique, often used at the beginning or end of a Qigong session.

One of the key benefits of the Golden Ball exercise is that it teaches the body how to feel and connect with Qi. As you stand in this position with relaxed focus, the body begins to open, subtle sensations of warmth, tingling, or pulsing may arise, and a sense of centeredness develops. With consistent practice, the Golden Ball helps to ground your energy, making it especially beneficial for those feeling anxious, scattered, or drained. It also strengthens the Dan Tian, the body's main energy storage center located in the lower abdomen, which plays a critical role in vitality and internal balance.

This exercise also improves postural alignment, as it encourages you to align the 18 key points of Qigong posture: feet rooted, spine lengthened, chest open, and head lifted lightly. The stillness of the posture gives the nervous system a chance to shift into a parasympathetic (rest–and–digest) state, promoting healing, clarity, and emotional calm.

Mentally and spiritually, the Golden Ball invites a meditative state of awareness. Visualizing a radiant ball of light between the hands can stimulate a deep connection with one's inner energy and even a sense of awe or peace. Some practitioners imagine the ball expanding and contracting with each breath or glowing with golden light that nourishes every cell of the body.

Though the Golden Ball requires no movement, it is a profoundly dynamic experience internally. Practicing it regularly, even for just 5–10 minutes a day, can lead to noticeable improvements in energy levels, focus, stress reduction, and emotional stability. In essence, it serves as a bridge between the physical and energetic realms, offering a simple yet powerful tool to harmonize body, mind, and spirit. As I'm building my YouTube channel as I write this, I don't have much Qigong at the moment. There are a plethora of Qigong masters and practitioners out there on YouTube, just plug in some of these keywords and have some fun! One of my Qigong teachers is JC Cox from Las Vegas. He runs the Golden Dragon Arts (www.BecomeQiGong.com) and you can find him on social media as well.

Tension and Relaxation

One of the core principles in Qigong is the deliberate use of tension and relaxation to guide energy, build strength, and release blockages within the body. While Qigong is often associated with slow, flowing movements and deep calm, the purposeful application of tension, followed by conscious release, plays a powerful role in cultivating both physical vitality and energetic harmony. This balance of opposites mirrors the Yin–Yang philosophy that underlies much of traditional Chinese medicine and martial arts.

In practice, tension in Qigong is not forced or excessive. Instead, it is light and intentional, designed to create structure, awareness, and connection. For example, when performing a movement like "Pushing the Wave" or "Spreading the Wings," the practitioner may briefly engage the muscles of the arms, legs, or core, as if resisting gentle pressure. This tension awakens the body's awareness, stimulates circulation, and engages the nervous system. Just as importantly, once that moment of effort passes, it is followed by a conscious softening, release, and relaxation, which allows the Qi to flow more freely and deeply.

This cycle of engage and release offers numerous benefits. Physically, it improves muscle tone, posture, and joint stability without the stress or fatigue often caused by high–impact exercise. By subtly engaging and then relaxing the muscles, the body becomes more fluid,

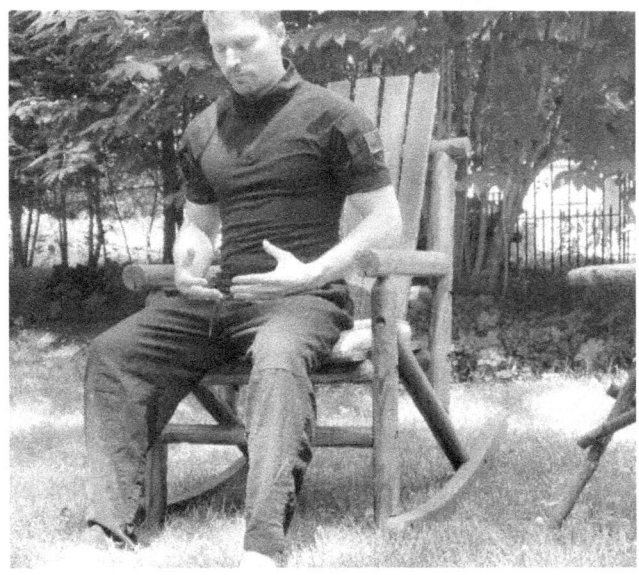

strong, and supple, while reducing tension held in areas like the neck, shoulders, and lower back.

Energetically, the rhythm of tension and relaxation acts like a pump for Qi, increasing the body's internal awareness and strengthening the pathways through which energy flows. This process also supports the lymphatic and circulatory systems, helping to clear out stagnant energy and toxins, while improving immunity and cellular function.

Mentally and emotionally, this practice trains the nervous system to move between alertness and calm. It teaches the practitioner how to let go, which is especially valuable in modern life where stress often lingers in the body long after a challenging event. By practicing this cycle regularly, the body learns that it is safe to release tension, which can have profound effects on stress management, anxiety, and trauma recovery.

On a deeper level, the technique of tension and relaxation can also become a form of emotional alchemy. Emotions, like energy, can get stuck when we hold too tightly to them, whether it's fear, anger, or sadness. In Qigong, using light tension to "bring up" awareness in the body, followed by gentle release, helps unravel these emotional knots in a safe and non-invasive way.

Over time, practicing tension and relaxation in Qigong develops a profound sensitivity to the body's inner signals. It allows you to feel more grounded, more in control, and more connected to your breath, your body, and your internal energy. It's not just about movement, it's about learning how to move through life with more ease, strength, and presence. Whether you're recovering from stress, seeking more vitality, or simply trying to reconnect with your body, this technique offers a deeply healing and empowering path.

Dan Tian: Understanding the Lower, Middle, and Upper Dan Tians

In Qigong and traditional Chinese medicine, the body has three main energy centers known as the Dan Tians or Dan Tiens (pronounced "dahn tee–en"), which means "elixir fields" or "energy centers." These are not physical organs, but energetic areas that store and process life force energy, or Qi. You can think of them like internal batteries or power centers that each relate to different aspects of our health and being: the body, heart, and mind.

The Lower Dan Tien is located in the lower belly, about two to three finger widths below the navel and a few inches inward. This is considered the foundation of all energy work. It stores your core life force, helps you feel grounded, and gives you physical vitality. If you've ever felt like you have no energy or feel "scattered," chances are your Lower Dan Tian needs some attention. Practicing Qigong, breathing into the belly, and grounding visualizations help recharge this area. It's closely connected to your root, stability, and physical health.

The Middle Dan Tian is located in the center of the chest, around the heart area. This center is related to emotions, compassion, relationships, and the breath. When you feel love, connection, or grief, it's the Middle Dan Tian that's being activated. A healthy Middle Dan Tian allows you to express feelings clearly, live with emotional balance, and develop kindness toward yourself and others. Heart–opening Qigong movements, breathwork, and forgiveness practices help nourish this center.

The Upper Dan Tian is located between the eyebrows, often called the "third eye." It governs mental clarity, intuition, insight, and spiritual awareness. When balanced, this center helps you think clearly, make wise decisions, and connect to a deeper sense of purpose. Practices like meditation, visualization, and stillness nourish the Upper Dan Tian. It's like your inner compass or antenna to higher awareness.

These three Dan Tians work together like a team. The Lower Dan Tian grounds you, the Middle Dan Tian connects you emotionally, and the Upper Dan Tian guides your mind and spirit. When all three are in harmony, you feel centered, energized, emotionally balanced, and mentally clear. Qigong helps us connect to and balance these energy centers so we can live a more healthy, peaceful, and aligned life.

1–10 QiGong Visualization Exercise

This is one of my favorite visualizations and I've done a lot of them! You can practice this either sitting or standing. If you're in a fatigued state, begin by sitting, and work your way up to standing as your strength improves. Over time, as you become more familiar with the practice, you can begin integrating proper posture and even incorporate Wu Ji stance into it. I'll guide you through the process as if you're standing but know that the same principles apply when sitting. At first, your posture doesn't need to be perfect, just focus on the basics.

Standing: Position your feet shoulder–width apart, or slightly wider if more comfortable. Keep your feet facing straight forward, flat on the ground with a subtle lift in the inner arches. Your knees should be soft—either slightly bent or neutral—but never locked. Keep your hips in a neutral position, your lower back relaxed, and your neck loose and aligned.

Sitting: Wear loose, natural, and comfortable clothing. Sit in a way that feels relaxed and grounded, don't sit stiffly like you're tied to a broomstick. Support your back if needed, such as by resting against the back of a chair.

In both positions, let your hands lay in front of your Lower Dan Tian (just below the navel) as if you're gently holding a volleyball–sized golden ball of light.

IMPORTANT NOTE:
REMEMBER TO BREATHE THROUGHOUT THE EXERCISE.
If you start feeling lightheaded or spaced out, gently bring your attention back to your lower belly and pause the exercise if needed.

Close your eyes and visualize yourself holding that golden ball of energy, part of the ball resting inside your belly. Now bring your attention down to your feet. Imagine tree roots extending from the soles of your feet, reaching into the Earth. There's no need to be technical, visualize it in whatever way feels right to you. Some see the roots going deep into the Earth's core, others just a few feet down.

Now, imagine Golden Life Force Energy rising up through those roots, entering through your feet, traveling up the inner legs, into your root center and core. From there, it flows up the back of the spine, over the top of the head, down the face, and down the front of the body forming a full energy circuit. This energy collects and begins to fill your Lower Dan Tian, steadily building and radiating from that center point. Eventually, it overflows, spreading through your entire body, until your whole being is glowing with golden energy.

Next, visualize the crown of your head gently opening, allowing Heavenly Energy to pour down into your body. This white, luminous energy flows in through the top of your head, mixing with the golden energy already within you.

Finally, imagine this radiant Golden–White Energy expanding beyond your body, filling your energy field. Start small, perhaps just a foot or two around you. As your awareness and energy increase with practice, you can gradually extend it out to its natural full size, which for many people is around 5 to 10 feet in all directions, forming a glowing sphere of energy surrounding your body.

This visualization is powerful, centering, and deeply restorative. It connects Heaven and Earth within you, grounding your energy while opening you to clarity, vitality, and peace.

I like to use this memory mnemonic to help me remember the steps for this exercise.
- 1 is Fun, try to make it fun!
- 2 is Shoe, from the lower Dan Tian, move attention to the feet.
- 3 is Tree, tree roots grow out of feet and into the Earth.

- 4 is Core, bring the golden divine light back up the legs and into the lower root core of the body, up the spine, over the head and down into the lower Dan Tian.
- 5 is Alive, feeling "Alive" with this golden energy.
- 6 is Thick, feeling the body filled up and "thick" with this energy.
- 7 is Heaven, heavenly white light coming down from "Heavens" into the crown and mixes with the Golden light filling up the body.
- 8 is Gate, like a gate opening from your body and shines and flows out into your energy field.
- 9 is Shine, your body and outside the body, your energy field is shining with this golden white light.
- 10 is do it again. You don't need to do this over again but try to stay consistent.

Pressure Point and Trigger Point Massage

When it comes to relieving anxiety and stress, the body holds several key pressure points that, when gently massaged, can help calm the nervous system, ease tension, and promote a sense of inner peace. You can use your thumb or middle finger, either are commonly used to apply pressure.

IMPORTANT NOTE:
The acupressure, acupuncture, and self–massage techniques shared in this book are for educational purposes only and are not a substitute for professional medical advice, diagnosis, or treatment. Always consult with a qualified healthcare provider before beginning any new practice, especially if you are pregnant, have a medical condition, or are recovering from an injury. Certain pressure points should be avoided during pregnancy or in specific health situations. Use these techniques mindfully and at your own discretion.

Yintang, located between the eyebrows and often referred to as the "third eye," is one of the most calming points on the body. Gently massaging this area can help soothe mental tension, reduce worry, and ease overthinking. It's a great point to use at the beginning of a relaxation routine or meditation practice.

GV 20 (Baihui) is located at the top of the head, in line with the tops of the ears. This point helps uplift the spirit, clear mental fog, and promote a sense of centeredness. It is especially useful when you feel disconnected or mentally scattered.

Heart 7 (Shenmen) is found on the pinky side of the wrist crease. Known as the "Spirit Gate," this point is commonly used for calming anxiety, promoting emotional balance, and supporting restful sleep. It's ideal during moments of emotional overwhelm or panic.

Pericardium 6 (Neiguan) is located about two to three finger-widths above the wrist on the inner forearm. This point is excellent for calming the heart, relieving chest tightness, and easing emotional distress. It also helps with anxiety-related nausea or upset stomach.

Kidney 1 (Yongquan) lies on the sole of the foot, about a third of the way down from the toes to the heel. This grounding point is especially useful when anxious thoughts feel overwhelming or when the energy in the body feels too "up" or scattered. It draws the energy downward, creating stability and calm.

Liver 3 (Taichong) is located on the top of the foot, in the space between the big toe and second toe. This point helps release built-up emotional tension, irritability, and internal frustration. It supports the smooth flow of energy throughout the body and mind.

Large Intestine 4 (Hegu) is found in the webbing between the thumb and index finger. It's a powerful point for releasing physical tension, especially in the head and neck, and is known for calming the nervous system. It should be avoided during pregnancy but is very effective for stress and anxiety relief.

Stomach 36 (Zusanli) is about four finger-widths below the kneecap, slightly to the outside of the shinbone. This point is excellent for boosting energy, supporting digestion, and reducing stress-related fatigue. It helps the body stay strong and resilient under pressure.

Bladder 10 (Tianzhu) is located at the base of the skull, about one inch out from the spine on either side. Massaging this point can help relieve neck tension, ease headaches, and calm the nervous system, especially when feeling mentally overworked or emotionally drained.

Conception Vessel 17 (CV17) is in the center of the chest, at the level of the heart. It is often called the "Sea of Tranquility" and is one of the best points for calming emotional turbulence. It also helps open the lungs and support deeper, more relaxed breathing during stress.

Gallbladder 21 (Jianjing) is located at the top of the shoulders, halfway between the base of the neck and the edge of the shoulder. This point holds a lot of physical tension and is useful for releasing built up stress in the upper body. It should be used with caution and avoided during pregnancy.

Anmian, or the "Peaceful Sleep Point," is found just behind the ear at the base of the skull. This point is excellent for calming the mind and promoting deep, restful sleep. It is especially helpful for people who experience racing thoughts, restlessness, or anxiety-related insomnia.

Stomach 36 (ST36), also known as **Zusanli**, is located about four finger-widths below the kneecap and one finger-width to the outside of the shinbone. Stimulating ST36 boosts energy, strengthens digestion, supports the immune system, and helps reduce stress and fatigue.

Using these points daily, even just for a few minutes, can become a powerful self-care practice for managing anxiety and maintaining emotional balance. Combined with deep breathing and mindful attention, they help restore calm, clarity, and a grounded sense of well-being.

Self-massage

This has been one of the most powerful practices in my life, and it holds great potential for many others as well. Use the same idea here as with the pressure points we just went over. Despite its simplicity, massage is often overlooked. Massage, in general, is a deeply rooted and ancient healing technique, practiced across countless cultures for thousands of years. While every culture has developed its own unique approach, the underlying principle remains the same: getting someone's hands, or your own, on your body to promote healing and relaxation.

When the body enters a state of fight or flight, tension builds up in the muscles, fascia, tissues, and even in deeper layers like the joints, organs, and meridians. A fear or stress response causes the body to contract, which restricts blood flow and impedes the natural circulation of energy. When this flow is blocked, it's as if the body's internal river has been dammed, and Qi and blood are no longer reaching the areas that need nourishment. Your system then becomes stagnant.

Massage works to break down this tension, releasing constriction and restoring the body's natural flow. You can think of stress and emotional tension like a dam in a river, blocking the water from reaching the fields or flowing into the ocean. When you begin to release that blockage, life energy and vitality can move freely again.

Ancient cultures, including those in Chinese and Thai traditions, carefully mapped out pressure points and trigger points, many of which we've already discussed. These pressure points offer particularly powerful benefits when stimulated through massage. Personally, I practice Thai massage, which often involves sustained downward pressure and passive stretching, folding the body into yoga-like postures to unlock deeply held tension.

But, since we're focusing on self–massage, let's stay grounded in what you can do with your own two hands. A great place to start is with the feet. There are countless YouTube videos on foot massage and reflexology, many of which I've learned from myself, alongside my formal study in Thai massage. The truth is, it doesn't have to be complicated or intimidating. It just takes a little time, presence, and attention. Even a few minutes of foot massage can ground your energy, calm your nervous system, and restore a sense of calm and well–being.

We won't be going into this in detail in this book, but it's worth mentioning that acupuncture and meridian therapy have been incredibly helpful for me personally, and for so many others around the world. These practices, rooted in Traditional Chinese Medicine (TCM), focus on restoring balance and flow to the body's energy system (your Qi or Chi).

Palming and Thumb Pressure

Using the flat soft palm of your hand, start applying pressure to the inside of your ankle, you can use one or both hands. Palming up to the inside of the knee and back down, take about one to two minutes for each leg. Lay flat on your back and use both thumbs on the back of the upper neck, massaging in circles with medium pressure. Try looking for the bladder 10 pressure point just below the ridge of the back of the skull and outside the ropey upper neck muscles.

Abdomen

I can't express the importance of this section enough! In both reflexology and traditional healing systems like Qigong and Ayurveda, the belly, particularly the area around the navel, is considered a central hub for emotional tension, digestion, and energy flow. This area also corresponds to the solar plexus, often associated with anxiety, fear, and emotional holding.

To begin, lie down or sit comfortably and place your hands gently on your abdomen. Using your fingertips or palms, massage around the navel in slow, clockwise circles, starting small and gradually widening the circles. Apply gentle pressure, enough to feel warmth and movement, but not so much that it causes discomfort. Breathe deeply and slowly as you do this, focusing your attention on the warmth of your hands and the rhythm of your breath.

This technique helps stimulate digestion, ease bloating or tension, and signal the body that it is safe to relax. More importantly, it helps release emotional stress held in the gut, where many people unconsciously store anxiety. Regular self–massage around the navel can improve emotional regulation, reduce stress and nervous tension, and promote a deep sense of grounding and calm. For enhanced effects, combine this practice with slow belly breathing or a calming essential oil like lavender or chamomile. Even just 5 minutes a day can make a noticeable difference in your mood and mental clarity.

Gentle abdominal massage, breathwork, nervous system regulation, and dietary support can all help bring the ICV back into balance. Some practitioners use specific manual techniques to reset the valve, and others address it through reflexology or acupuncture. Addressing underlying emotional stress, calming the nervous system, and supporting digestion are essential steps in restoring proper ileocecal valve function and improving overall well–being.

Ileocecal Valve

The ileocecal valve (ICV) is a small but important valve located between the small intestine (ileum) and the large intestine (cecum). Its main job is to control the flow of digested food from the small intestine into the large intestine, and to prevent backflow of waste. When functioning properly, it helps maintain healthy digestion and keeps bacteria in the right places. However, when the valve malfunctions, either staying open or closed too long, it can lead to a range of digestive issues, such as bloating, gas, constipation, diarrhea, abdominal pain, and even referred pain in areas like the lower back or shoulder.

What many people don't realize is that stress, anxiety, and PTSD can significantly affect the ileocecal valve through the vagus nerve. The Vagus nerve controls all the "valves and "sphincters" in the body. The digestive system is closely tied to the nervous system through the gut–brain axis, meaning emotional stress has a direct impact on digestive function. When someone is living in a prolonged fight–or–flight state (as is often the case with PTSD or chronic anxiety), the body deprioritizes digestion. This can lead to tension and dysfunction in the muscles around the digestive tract, including the ileocecal valve.

When stress is high, the valve may become spasmodic or sluggish, leading to poor elimination, the buildup of toxins, and further gut inflammation. This not only affects physical comfort but can worsen mood, increase fatigue, and heighten emotional sensitivity, creating a feedback loop where gut dysfunction contributes to anxiety and vice versa. This is why many people with anxiety or PTSD also report chronic digestive problems.

Temples

We all know the temples. Use light to medium pressure with your thumbs, or one to two fingers and massage in a circular motion. Relax the eyes while taking a few deep slow breaths. Massage for a minute or two.

Acupuncture

Acupuncture involves the gentle insertion of ultra–fine needles into specific points along the body's meridian pathways. These meridians are like energetic highways that connect different organs and systems, likened to rivers and waterways. When energy becomes blocked, deficient, or excessive in certain areas, it can lead to physical pain, emotional imbalance, or fatigue. By stimulating these points, acupuncture helps to clear blockages, regulate the nervous system, and promote natural healing.

Think of pressure points like natural water springs with water coming up from under the ground and sprouting out onto the earth's surface or on the bottom of a river or lakebed. Pressure points are special spots that when triggered, massaged or needled, can reach into the body in a deeper and more supportive way, triggering the meridians and reaching deeper into the organs and energy centers like the Dan Tians. One of my acupuncturists once told me that one foundational aspect in helping a person is to bring the deficient UP and bring the excessive DOWN. Now, there's a lot more to it than that but that was a good piece of wisdom.

All in all, go get some acupuncture! Ask around and read reviews, some acupuncturists are different than others. Some practice in a more "intense way," others are gentler. Some use herbs as part of the practice, which can be great, but it's often much more expensive. Also ask if you get acupuncture as part of your insurance. After receiving treatment, this is something that works over a period of days to a week. Since acupuncture shifts internal energies and allows blood to flow, it can take some time for the body to come into homeostasis (balance). Make sure you drink fluids and electrolytes after receiving a session, and do the same with meridian therapy, pressure points and massage.

Meridian Therapy

Meridian therapy is also closely tied to self-massage and includes techniques like acupressure, cupping, and moxibustion. Each work along the same principles, but may use heat, touch, or suction instead of needles. These therapies can be especially beneficial for people dealing with stress, anxiety, chronic pain, digestive issues, hormonal imbalance, sleep disturbances, and more.

What's powerful about these methods is that they don't just treat symptoms, they aim to realign the entire system, helping the body return to a natural state of balance. I've personally found that acupuncture and meridian therapy not only relieve tension in the body but also help regulate emotions, calm the mind, and boost overall vitality. Even if you're someone who's a bit skeptical of energy–based practices, countless people (me included) have experienced real, tangible benefits from them. This is another area where pretty much every culture has some form of understanding of "meridians" or "energy lines." They've been called many things. In Thai Yoga/Thai Massage, they are called "ley" lines. As far as this book goes, I focus on self-massage or asking your significant other or a friend to do some basic massage.

While we won't go deep into the theory or history here, it's something I always recommend exploring further for improving your wellbeing and building a healthier lifestyle.

Takeaways from Chapter 9:

- Qi Gong, Chi Gong, Chi Kung, and Ki Kung all refer to the same ancient practice, which translates loosely to "energy work" or "breath work." At its core, Qi Gong is about moving energy and blood through the body to create healing, balance, and vitality.
- Daily Practice: you can easily add Qi Gong into your daily routine. It serves not only as gentle exercise but also as a powerful tool for mindfulness, mental focus, and calming the nervous system. Think of it as a "cool down" for your energy and your mind.
- Purge–Tonify–Regulate is one of the foundational principles of Qi Gong and Chinese medicine.
    - *Purge* what no longer serves you—physically, emotionally, mentally, and even in your environment. Clean the clutter in all areas.
    - *Tonify* by strengthening yourself, your energy, your physical constitution, and your sense of purpose.
    - *Regulate* by allowing things to settle and return to flow. When we stop over controlling, our body and mind often know how to find balance on their own. But sometimes, we need to purge and tonify first before regulation can naturally occur.
- Relaxation in Layers — let the body soften. Let the breath slow. Let the mind loosen its grip. Let your energy settle. And finally, allow your spirit to relax, open, and guide you more fully. This is where true healing begins.
- Energy Sensitivity is real. If you're energy sensitive like I am (and like many others I've worked with), energy work can have a profound impact on your health and quality of life. Don't dismiss it until you've tried it—it may become one of your most powerful healing tools.
- Yin and Yang Awareness — Understanding Yin and Yang even at a basic level can radically improve your approach to life. It helps you recognize imbalance and move toward harmony. Remember, *balance* is everything. It's the sweet spot. The half–court swish. The "in–the–zone" flow state. Too many people

bounce from one extreme to the next, chasing perfection in either direction. But balance? That's where the magic happens.

Chapter 10
Nature, Exercise and Martial Arts

"The happiness of your life depends upon the quality of your thoughts."
— *Marcus Aurelius*

Let's talk about nature. The healing power of nature offers a profound way to reduce anxiety and alleviate stress. Spending time in natural settings, whether it's a forest, beach, park, garden or even your backyard, has been shown to lower cortisol, the body's primary stress hormone. Being in nature can help calm the nervous system, which encourages a state of relaxation. This effect is often accompanied by reduced blood pressure and improved heart rate, fostering a sense of calm and wellbeing.

Natural environments also have a unique ability to engage our senses, allowing us to reconnect with the present moment and distance ourselves from the distractions and pressures of daily life. The sounds of birds, the rustle of leaves, and the sight of natural landscapes can help shift our focus away from anxiety–inducing thoughts, promoting a sense of peace. Additionally, exposure to natural sunlight boosts vitamin D levels, which is essential for mood regulation and mental health. Regular time outdoors can help increase feelings of happiness and reduce symptoms of depression, making it an effective, accessible form of selfcare.

In Japan, the concept of "nature bathing" is known as *shinrin–yoku*, which literally translates to "forest bath." It refers to the practice of immersing oneself in nature, especially in forests, to promote mental, physical, and emotional wellbeing. The term was coined in the 1980s by the Japanese Ministry of Agriculture, Forestry, and Fisheries as a way to highlight the health benefits of spending time in natural environments.

This practice encourages individuals to slow down and engage their senses fully with the natural surroundings, whether it's the smell of the trees, the sound of rustling leaves, or the feel of the ground beneath your feet. Research has shown that *shinrin–yoku* can lower stress, improve mood, boost the immune system, and increase feelings of relaxation and calm.

It's not just about being outdoors; it's about being present in nature, taking time to breathe deeply, and disconnecting from the fast-paced, technology driven world. The idea is that nature has a therapeutic power that can restore balance and improve overall health. It's quite popular in Japan and has gained attention in other parts of the world as well.

Physical activity in nature, such as walking or hiking, releases endorphins, the body's natural mood enhancing chemicals, which can reduce feelings of anxiety. Nature also encourages mindfulness and a slower pace, helping to quiet the mind and provide a mental break from stress. This combination of sensory stimulation, physical movement, and quietude makes nature a powerful ally in improving mental health and fostering resilience against stress and anxiety.

To begin getting the benefits of nature, start by walking a minimum of 20 to 30 min a day 4 times a week. Depending on your physical ability and health, try to walk more and start power walking. One of my old psychologists once told me, "20 minutes of walking a day is good for your mental health, 30 minutes a day is good for your physical health."

Exercise and cardio turn on the burners in your body. This then improves your blood and circulation, helps your organs work better, takes out the garbage, and opens up the glands to release natural mood enhancing endorphins, which activate our opiate receptors!

IMPORTANT NOTE:
If you have a history of chronic health problems, chronic fatigue, other similar issues or haven't exercised at all in a long time, **I don't want you to be doing any high or even moderate cardio.** This will spike cortisol and will likely cause more burnout. You want to be doing low impact and light movements. Such as yoga, Qigong, Taichi, walking, light calisthenics, or light martial arts (learn the technical martial arts which is what I love to teach, NOT grappling to start with).

Getting More Sunshine

Getting morning sunlight, especially within the first hour of waking, is one of the simplest and most effective ways to support overall mental and physical health. When natural light enters the eyes (without sunglasses), it signals the brain to regulate your circadian rhythm, the internal clock that controls your sleep–wake cycle. This light exposure helps the brain reduce melatonin (the sleep hormone) and increase cortisol and serotonin, boosting mood, focus, and energy throughout the day. We need some cortisol in the morning and during the daytime for healthy energy levels. Cortisol is part of what helps us feel awake and active! When cortisol gets over stimulated because of too much anxiety and stress, that's when we get too out of balance.

Daytime sunlight also stimulates the production of vitamin D through the skin, which plays a key role in immune function, bone health, hormone balance, and mental well–being. Low levels of vitamin D have been linked to depression, anxiety, and PTSD, making regular sun exposure an important part of emotional healing and nervous system support. For those with stress–related issues, trauma, or fatigue, getting daily morning sunlight can help regulate mood, improve sleep quality, and restore a sense of natural rhythm and balance to both body and mind.

Most people typically don't get vitamin D in the morning time but instead get sunlight from around 10 a.m. to about 4:30 p.m. However, we get different benefits from morning sunlight versus daytime sunlight. You want to get some time in the sun *without* sunscreen, as that blocks vitamin D. You don't want to burn your skin so use common sense. I'm a fair lighter skinned individual and I like to get about 20 to 30 minutes of direct sunlight on my skin and on as much of my skin as possible. After that I may put on clothing to cover up, or put on non-toxic sunscreen, or just go in the shade if I'm outside swimming or doing other things. Certain parts of the body absorb more sunlight than others. These parts are higher in nerve endings as well so that is a correlation. This includes the palms of the hands and feet, armpits, inner arms and the groin region. Keep this in mind when you're outside enjoying the sunlight.

Getting More Exercise

Exercise plays a crucial role in regulating the body's stress response, particularly for those dealing with PTSD, anxiety, and panic. One of the key ways it helps is by **burning off excess adrenaline and cortisol**, the primary stress hormones that flood the body during moments of heightened fear or anxiety. When someone experiences PTSD or panic attacks, their nervous system often remains in a hyperactive state, leading to chronic tension, restlessness, and difficulty relaxing. Physical movement provides an outlet for this built-up energy, helping to regulate the nervous system and bring the body back to a state of balance.

Additionally, exercise helps **burn off excess glucose** in the blood and tissues. During stress, the body releases glucose as an immediate energy source, preparing for a fight–or–flight response. However, if this energy is not used, it remains in the bloodstream, potentially leading to blood sugar imbalances, insulin resistance, and increased inflammation. Engaging in physical activity helps process and utilize this excess glucose, stabilizing energy levels and reducing the risk of metabolic issues.

Once again, if you have been chronically ill or fatigued for an extended period, moderate to high-intensity cardio and exercise are *not* appropriate. This fact is often overlooked by fitness influencers, doctors, and even many health experts. I've made this mistake in my own past, pushing through when my body wasn't ready. For individuals in this state, exercise can actually be harmful, triggering flare-ups, worsening fatigue, and requiring extended recovery time.

The solution? Focus on low-impact, gentle movements that support healing rather than depleting it. As discussed throughout this book, practices like yoga, Qi Gong, Tai Chi, slow walking, light calisthenics, gardening, mindful housework, and even playing calmly with your kids can all provide valuable physical stimulation without overstressing the body. Light martial arts training, focusing more on form, balance, breath, and the *art* itself rather than intensity, can also be a powerful option.

Even mental strain, like excessive thinking or overanalyzing, can be too much for someone in a depleted state. That was true for me as well. You'll need to become more aware of your body's signals and respect your current limits while gently building your strengths.

Feel free to visit my YouTube channel (@WasenshiDo), where I've created a 30-Day Martial Arts for Beginners series designed specifically to support balance, focus, and gentle progress. You'll find techniques and exercises to help restore energy and confidence at a pace that works with your body, not against it.

Another major benefit of exercise is its ability to **reduce inflammation**. Chronic stress, PTSD, and anxiety are often linked to increased inflammation throughout the body, which can contribute to a range of health issues, including joint pain, digestive problems, and weakened immune function. Exercise helps counteract this by promoting circulation, improving immune function, and triggering the release of anti-inflammatory compounds. Movement also increases the production of **endorphins and serotonin**, which not only reduces pain perception but also improves mood, making exercise one of the most natural and effective ways to support both mental and physical health. Whether it's high-intensity training, weightlifting, yoga, or simple walking, regular physical activity is a powerful tool for managing stress, improving metabolic health, and fostering long-term wellbeing.

From the view of Taoism and Chinese medicine, panic and anxiety disorders are often seen as Yin imbalances, too much stillness, overthinking, internal pressure, and not enough outward energy or movement. Yin represents coolness, rest, and inward focus, which are important, but when there's too much Yin and not enough balance, it can lead to emotional stagnation, fear, and a feeling of being stuck in your head or body. In simple terms, the system gets too slow, heavy, and quiet on the inside.

To bring things back into balance, the body needs more Yang energy, movement, warmth, sunlight, activity, and motivation. Yang is the energy that gets things moving again. Getting outside in the morning light, walking, stretching, practicing martial arts or Qigong, or even just doing chores with intention can help shift you back into flow. These aren't just "good habits" they're literally helping your energy move and rebalance.

On a more physical level, exercise also ties into your mitochondria, the little engines in your cells that create ATP, aka energy. When you move your body and get sunlight, you help your mitochondria work better by giving you more energy, sharper thinking, and a stronger sense of calm. To tie this into the nutrition section, mitochondrial health is very much a Yang function, it's about power, drive, and inner fire. So, when you feel overwhelmed, stuck, or anxious, sometimes what you need most isn't more stillness, but the right kind of gentle action to wake up your inner energy system.

Calisthenics, or bodyweight training, is one of the best forms of exercise for overall health and mental well-being. Since it doesn't require equipment, it can be done anywhere, making it an accessible and effective way to build strength, improve mobility, and boost endurance. Movements like pushups, squats, pull-ups, and lunges engage multiple muscle groups at once, helping to increase coordination and functional strength that translates into everyday activities.

Beyond physical benefits, calisthenics has a powerful impact on mental health, especially for those dealing with anxiety, PTSD, and stress–related conditions. One of the key reasons is that it helps burn off excess adrenaline and cortisol, the stress hormones that flood the body during panic, fear, or trauma responses. Many people with PTSD or anxiety feel stuck in a state of heightened alertness, where their nervous system is constantly on edge. Calisthenics provides a natural outlet for this excess energy, helping the body return to a more relaxed state.

Additionally, engaging in bodyweight training regulates blood sugar and reduces inflammation, which is often linked to anxiety and stress. Exercise also triggers the release of endorphins and serotonin, the body's natural feel–good chemicals, which help stabilize mood, reduce tension, and promote a sense of calm. Since calisthenics requires focus, breath control, and body awareness, it can be a form of mindfulness in motion, grounding the mind in the present moment.

Another advantage is that mastering bodyweight movements builds confidence and resilience. Seeing progress in strength, flexibility, and endurance can be empowering, especially for those overcoming personal struggles. Whether it's doing a first pull–up, holding a handstand, or simply feeling stronger in daily life, calisthenics proves that growth is possible with consistency. For anyone dealing with PTSD, anxiety, or chronic stress, bodyweight training is a simple yet highly effective way to regain control of both the body and mind.

Martial arts

Marial arts aren't just about throwing punches, flipping people over, or looking cool in a "Keikogi" (Gi uniform). They're one of the most effective, primal, and oddly therapeutic ways to **punch anxiety and PTSD in the face** (metaphorically speaking or literally speaking, if you're working with a heavy bag). Unlike hitting the gym and staring at yourself in the mirror while pretending to know how to use a kettlebell, martial arts force you to be fully present, using your body and mind together in a way that's both intense and meditative.

One of the biggest benefits of martial arts for anxiety and PTSD is that it **burns off excess adrenaline and cortisol**, those lovely stress hormones that turn you into a jittery, overthinking mess. When the fight–or–flight system is constantly firing (which, let's be honest, is exhausting), martial arts give you a safe and controlled outlet to channel that energy. Whether it's kicking, striking, grappling, or even just drilling techniques over and over, your body learns to release tension instead of holding onto it like an unpaid intern clinging to their first job.

Then there's the breathing. You can't hyperventilate mid sparring, well, you *can*, but you won't last long! Martial arts naturally teach breath control, body awareness, and focus, which are all things that help calm the nervous system. The deep breathing and rhythmic movement act as a moving meditation, helping to regulate emotions and keep you from overanalyzing every possible worst–case scenario in life (because let's face it, anxiety loves doing that).

And let's not forget the confidence boost. If you've ever dealt with PTSD or anxiety, you know how easy it is to feel powerless. Martial arts flip the script. You learn how to move with intention, control your reactions, and trust your body again. There's something wildly empowering about realizing you're capable of defending yourself, or even just seeing progress in your training. Whether you finally land that perfect roundhouse kick or simply learn to stay calm under pressure, martial arts rebuild mental resilience in a way that therapy alone sometimes can't.

On top of all that, martial arts build a sense of community, something that's crucial for anyone struggling with anxiety or PTSD. You train with others, develop mutual respect, and form bonds with people who, let's be real, *also* probably started training to handle their own internal battles. It's a space where you can work through struggles without judgment, where nobody cares about your past, just how well you show up on the mat.

So, whether you're dealing with stress, anxiety, or just need a *socially acceptable* way to hit things, martial arts are one of the best investments you can make in your mind and body. And if nothing else, you'll at least develop some cool moves for when someone cuts you off in traffic... just kidding. Mostly.

Connection Through Martial Arts

Martial arts are like a full–body Wi–Fi signal booster for your brain and awareness, it strengthens the connection between mind and body, making you more alert, reactive, and in tune with your surroundings. Unlike traditional workouts that focus on isolated movements, martial arts require constant adaptation, quick decision–making, and coordination, all of which forge stronger neural pathways between your brain and muscles. Every time you block, strike, evade, or counter, your brain is processing information at high speed, sending signals to your body to move efficiently while maintaining balance and precision.

One of the key ways martial arts improve brain function is through neuroplasticity, the brain's ability to create and strengthen new neural connections. Learning a new technique, refining movement patterns, or adjusting to an unpredictable opponent forces the brain to problem solve in real time. This enhances reaction speed, memory, and overall cognitive function. It's like turning your brain into a well–trained strategist that operates on instinct while still staying sharp and focused.

Beyond raw cognitive improvement, martial arts develop body awareness, also known as proprioception, which is the ability to sense where your body is in space. When training, you learn how to move with control, how to adjust your weight for balance, and how to read subtle cues from your environment or opponent. This heightened sense of awareness translates beyond the dojo or gym and into everyday life, making you more present, mindful, and aware of your surroundings.

Martial arts also strengthen the connection between breath, movement, and focus, reinforcing mental clarity and emotional regulation. Controlled breathing helps calm the nervous system, while precise movements demand concentration. Over time, this constant practice of mindfulness in motion rewires the brain to stay calm under pressure, react efficiently, and maintain control in both physical and emotional situations.

At its core, martial arts aren't just about learning how to fight, it's about mastering yourself. It sharpens the brain, deepens awareness, and creates a level of mind–body harmony that extends into all areas of life. Whether you're in the middle of a sparring match, navigating a stressful situation, or simply walking down the street, your brain and awareness are working together at a higher level—ready, focused, and fully engaged with the world around you.

There's an old saying: "martial arts isn't just about defeating bandits and bad guys, it's about defeating diseases and disorders." Looking at it another way is that martial arts help defeat both external threats (opponents) and internal struggles (illness, stress, mental disorders). This philosophy is deeply ingrained in martial arts culture. It's a powerful way of thinking about martial arts as a **holistic practice**, not just a fighting system.

Marial Arts Techniques

One of the most seemingly simple, yet powerful techniques is the focus point technique. Just pick an object or spot in the distance from where you are, and lightly focus on this object, try it for 10, 20 and then 30 seconds before working your way up to several minutes. An advanced practice would be doing this for 5 minutes or more. Be very still, keep the eyes soft. And, no moving, just breathing and blinking. Relax the face, the jaw and eyes and adopt a relaxed light focus. Don't overstrain your mind. Place the book down and see how long you can go!

Punching a bag, boxing, and engaging in controlled sparring offer powerful psychological and mental health benefits that go beyond just physical fitness. These activities provide a safe and focused outlet for releasing built–up tension, frustration, anger, or anxiety—emotions that, if left unexpressed, can linger in the body and lead to mental and emotional imbalances. The act of striking something with intention helps discharge adrenaline and cortisol, the body's primary stress hormones, creating a sense of relief, clarity, and calm afterward.

Boxing and bag work also sharpen mental focus and present–moment awareness, which helps quiet overthinking and redirect energy into purposeful action. It becomes a form of moving meditation where the mind must stay sharp, reactive, and aware of breath and body position. This intense focus has been shown to improve mood, reduce symptoms of depression, and increase confidence and self–efficacy (the belief that you can take control and protect yourself).

Sparring, when practiced respectfully and with proper guidance, helps develop emotional regulation, resilience, and self–control. It challenges you to stay calm under pressure, manage fear and anxiety, and make decisions with clarity and discipline, even when your adrenaline is high. For people with PTSD, trauma, or anxiety, these practices can help rebuild trust in the body, create a sense of safety, and support nervous system regulation.

Overall, striking and sparring practices offer a therapeutic blend of release, empowerment, and focus, helping the mind process emotion, sharpen awareness, and restore a sense of inner strength and balance.

The Five Elements in Martial Arts

Earth – Structure, Stability, Foundation
Physical: rooting, stance work, base strength, and balance. Earth is the

stability in your legs and core that grounds every technique.
Mental: discipline, patience, endurance. The Earth element teaches resilience and remaining calm under pressure.
Training Application: focus on stances (Kiba–dachi, Zenkutsu–dachi), slow kata, balance drills, low kicks, and groundwork to cultivate this element.
Live It: patience, resilience, quiet strength. Earth teaches you to endure, to stabilize, to hold your ground even when life feels chaotic.

Water – Adaptability, Flow, Timing
Physical: circular movements, joint locks, transitions, throws. Water is about yielding and redirecting force (Aikido–like flow).
Mental: emotional intelligence, intuition, adaptability. Staying soft yet sharp.
Training Application: practice grappling, redirection, rolling, escape drills, and partner sensitivity exercises to embody water's energy.
Live It: be open, emotionally aware, and flexible in the mind. Water doesn't resist change, it becomes it. Too much rigidity and it breaks. Water bends and keeps flowing.

Fire – Power, Intensity, Explosiveness
Physical: strikes, kiais, explosive movements, high–intensity drills. Fire is the *yang*, the spirit and flame behind the technique.
Mental: courage, motivation, assertiveness, inner drive. Fire fuels the will to fight and transform.
Training Application: striking drills, sparring, HIIT–style martial workouts, pad work, and yelling (kiai) to engage the fire element.
Live It: purpose, passion, courage. When your Fire is healthy, you act with conviction not aggression, be an assertive presence. Fire without control is destruction. Fire with discipline is power.

Air/Wind – Speed, Breath, Lightness
Physical: footwork, breathing, evasion, quick changes in direction. Air is the whisper before the storm, the grace, agility, and reaction time.
Mental: clarity, focus, calm awareness. Mastering breathing and staying light in spirit.
Training Application: breathwork, light–footed drills, evasions, fast

reflex combos, speed and reaction training.
Live It: mental clarity, calm awareness, a mind that sees but doesn't get stuck. Breathe into life like you breathe into your techniques. You can't hold the wind. You can only move with it.

Ether/Spirit – Awareness, Connection, Higher Purpose
Physical: meditation, internal arts (Qi Gong, Tai Chi), stillness in movement, presence. Ether links all other elements.
Mental/Emotional: compassion, mindfulness, spiritual intent. Fighting for something greater than ego—service, self–mastery.
Training Application: practice stillness, mindfulness, visualization, kata with intention, meditative breathing, and bowing rituals. This is the soul of the martial path.
Live It: compassion, humility, connection. Ether reminds us that the martial path is not about domination, it's about evolution. The most powerful warrior is the one who knows peace.

Allow some of this knowledge and wisdom to slowly seep into your daily life and practice. You don't need to force it, just stay open. Over time, it will begin to make more sense. You'll start to see how it connects to everything around you. The more you live it, the more it becomes part of you, and the more interesting, meaningful, and grounded life becomes.

Kettlebells

These are an incredibly versatile, efficient and effective training tool that offers a unique combination of strength, endurance, mobility, and cardiovascular benefits. Unlike traditional weights, the shape and handle of a kettlebell allow for dynamic movements that engage multiple muscle groups at once, improving functional strength and coordination. Exercises like swings, snatches, and Turkish get–ups challenge the body in ways that dumbbells and barbells often do not, promoting better grip strength, core stability, and explosive power. The constant need to stabilize the weight as it moves builds resilience in the joints and improves overall balance.

Kettlebell training also provides an intense cardiovascular workout, increasing heart rate and endurance while simultaneously developing muscle. This makes it an excellent choice for time-efficient workouts, allowing people to build strength and burn fat in a short period. Additionally, kettlebells are easy to store and require minimal space, making them a practical option for home workouts. Whether used for strength training, conditioning, or flexibility, kettlebells are a powerful tool that enhances athletic performance, prevents injury, and supports overall physical health.

Martial Arts and General Techniques to do Consistently

I'm not pushing you to do all of these every day, especially if you are dealing with Chronic Fatigue Syndrome/Myalgic Encephalomyelitis. But pick a few or a handful to start and do them consistently. Shoot for 10 minutes a day or so.

Pushups

These are a simple and efficient, yet powerful exercise that strengthen the upper body, core, and stability muscles. They primarily work the chest, shoulders, and triceps, while also engaging the core and lower back for support. Regular pushups improve overall strength, enhance posture, and increase endurance. They also promote better shoulder stability and mobility, which is essential for daily movements and athletic performance. Since pushups can be modified in various ways, from knee pushups to advanced variations like archer or one-arm pushups, they are a versatile bodyweight exercise that benefits people at all fitness levels. Make sure you keep your elbows tucked in to protect the shoulders and engage your core to prevent dumping/sinking in the lower back.

Squats

These are one of the best full-body movements for building leg strength, mobility, and overall power. They target the quadriceps, hamstrings, glutes, and lower back, while also activating the core to maintain balance and stability. Squats improve flexibility in the hips and ankles, making everyday activities like walking, bending, and lifting easier. Additionally, they help boost metabolism by engaging large muscle groups, leading to better endurance and fat–burning potential. Whether performed with body weight, dumbbells, or a barbell, squats are essential for building lower body strength and functional movement. Squat stretching is one of my favorites. Squat with legs a bit wider and place forearms on the inner thighs. Be careful of the groin here! I like to just push lightly back and forth and get a little spinal twist in at the same time.

Hanging from a Bar

Also known as passive or active hanging, is an excellent way to decompress the spine, improve grip strength, and enhance shoulder mobility. This movement helps counteract the negative effects of prolonged sitting and poor posture by allowing the spine to stretch and realign naturally. It also strengthens the forearms, wrists, and shoulder stabilizers, which are essential for injury prevention and upper body strength. Regularly incorporating hanging into a routine can improve overall flexibility, reduce shoulder tightness, and serve as a foundation for exercises like pull-ups and climbing. Proceed to do some pull-ups if you feel strong!

Inversions

This is where the head is lower than the heart, providing multiple circulatory, nervous system, and mobility benefits. They help increase blood flow to the brain, improving focus, mood, and cognitive function. Inversions stimulate the lymphatic system, aiding in detoxification and reducing inflammation. Additionally, they relieve spinal compression, making them beneficial for people who experience back pain or tightness. Whether done through headstands, handstands, or simple movements like legs–up–the–wall, inversions help improve balance, core strength, and relaxation by activating the parasympathetic nervous system.

Bouncing

Whether through light jumping, rebounding on a trampoline, or even quick foot movements, bouncing stimulates the lymphatic system, which helps flush out toxins and improve immune function. This movement also enhances circulation, joint flexibility, and coordination, making it an excellent way to wake up the body and boost energy levels. Additionally, bouncing strengthens the calves, ankles, and lower leg muscles, which are crucial for balance and injury prevention. Even short bursts of bouncing can help improve cardiovascular health and stimulate a sense of lightness and agility.

Stances

Pick a few stances to do for a minute or two. Start with horse stance or a defensive/front angle style stance. Horse stance is where you widen your stance little more than shoulder width and bend your knees with your feet pointing forward. Defensive stance is where you step back in a straight line with your right foot and then step back the left foot to the right about one to two feet while bending the knees. I recommend watching my stances video on my YouTube Channel @WasenshiDo to learn more. You can hold these stances or be active in them and move slightly back and forth. Watch those knees and don't extend the knees past the toes.

Balance

This practice is as simple as it sounds—balancing on one foot—but the benefits go far beyond physical stability. To start, just lift one foot off the ground and hold it out in front of you for about 30 seconds, then switch to the other side. It may seem basic, but even this small movement engages the deep stabilizing muscles throughout the body, especially in the ankles, legs, hips, and core. Over time, it helps correct postural imbalances and strengthens each side of the spine individually, promoting better overall alignment and body awareness.

On a deeper level, balancing exercises like this one are incredibly beneficial for mental health and brain function. Balancing requires focused attention, which pulls your mind into the present moment and acts as a form of active mindfulness. This improves concentration, coordination, and neural communication between the brain and body. As you develop this skill, the brain adapts by forming new neural pathways, which is great for neuroplasticity, your brain's ability to grow and change.

For those struggling with anxiety or stress, balance exercises can also help regulate the nervous system. They engage the vestibular system, which contributes to spatial orientation and a sense of groundedness. When you feel physically stable, the mind naturally feels calmer and more in control. Simple as it is, balancing on one foot is a powerful tool for building both physical resilience and mental clarity, all from just a few minutes of focused practice each day.

Shadow boxing

Shadow boxing is another deceptively simple practice that delivers a wide range of physical and mental benefits. It involves throwing punches, movements, and footwork in the air as if you're facing an imaginary opponent. While it may look like just punching the air, shadow boxing is a full–body, full–mind workout that improves coordination, speed, balance, and cardiovascular health, all without any equipment.

From a physical perspective, shadow boxing strengthens the shoulders, arms, core, and legs, while improving agility, posture, and spatial awareness. It also trains the body to move with purpose and fluidity, helping to develop muscle memory and refine technique. Because it's low–impact, it's accessible to almost everyone and can be done anywhere—from a living room to a quiet outdoor space.

On the mental health side, shadow boxing is a powerful way to release tension, reduce anxiety, and build confidence. The movement demands focus and presence, drawing your attention away from racing thoughts and into your breath, rhythm, and body. This makes it a form of moving meditation, where you're practicing mindfulness through motion. The act of throwing controlled punches—even without contact—allows you to channel emotions like frustration, anger, or stress in a safe and empowering way.

Neurologically, shadow boxing stimulates the brain through visualization, decision making, and timing, which supports cognitive sharpness and neuroplasticity. You're not just moving, you're strategizing, imagining, and reacting, even if it's all in your head. This dynamic interaction between body and mind builds mental agility, emotional resilience, and a strong mind–body connection.

In short, shadow boxing isn't just for fighters, it's for anyone who wants to feel stronger, more focused, and more grounded. Whether used as a warm–up, a workout, or a stress relief practice, it's a fast, free, and effective way to boost both physical vitality and mental clarity.

Spinal twists with punching

Spinal twists with punching combine two powerful movements into one dynamic and energizing practice. As you twist your torso from side to side and throw controlled punches, you're engaging not only the arms and shoulders, but also the core, spine, hips, and nervous system. This type of movement improves mobility and strength in the spine, increases rotational power, and helps to loosen up stiffness caused by prolonged sitting or stress.

Physically, this movement builds strength and flexibility through the midsection, activating the obliques, lower back, and hips while also encouraging proper spinal alignment. The twisting action gently compresses and decompresses the spine and internal organs, promoting better circulation, digestion, and detoxification. The addition of punches trains the upper body, builds cardiovascular endurance, and improves coordination and balance.

Mentally and emotionally, spinal twists with punching offer a unique way to release pent–up energy and bring the body into an alert, yet focused state. The rhythmic motion of twisting and striking helps regulate the nervous system, encouraging the body to shift out of "fight or flight" and into a more balanced, responsive state. The movement is grounding, empowering, and emotionally clearing—especially helpful for those managing anxiety, tension, or residual emotional stress.

From a brain–health perspective, this combo movement enhances cross–body coordination and bilateral integration, meaning both sides of the brain and body are working together. This is excellent for improving mental clarity, focus, and neural communication, which can sharpen reflexes and calm mental overactivity at the same time.

In short, spinal twists with punching offer a blend of mobility, strength, emotional release, and cognitive stimulation. It's an ideal movement for warming up, shaking off stress, or re–centering yourself during the day. Simple, effective, and energizing, this practice helps you build a strong body, a flexible spine, and a more focused, balanced mind.

In conclusion, there is real power in consistency. It's one of the most challenging things for people to maintain, yet it's often the very thing that creates lasting change. Even the simplest acts—like taking a daily walk in the sun, breathing deeply, or standing barefoot on the earth—can have profound effects when done consistently. These small habits, done regularly, put you a step ahead of the majority who wait for motivation rather than build momentum.

Try making your walk a morning ritual to help reset your circadian rhythm, you'll likely notice your mood, energy, and focus start to improve. Think about it this way: what would happen if you only ate one meal the entire week? Unless you're an advanced fasting expert, your body would likely rebel. Just like nutrition, your body and nervous system need consistent rhythms and inputs to feel safe, strong, and balanced. Consistency isn't just a nice idea, it's the foundation for real transformation.

Takeaways from Chapter 10:

- Spending time in nature—often called "nature bathing"—is one of the most powerful antidotes to stress and anxiety. Immersing yourself in natural environments helps calm the nervous system and reset your inner balance. Walking, even for just 5 minutes to start, is incredibly important for both mental and physical health. Over time, try to build up to 20 to 30 minutes of walking consistently, especially outdoors.
- Sunshine is essential to every aspect of our wellbeing. A few responsible sunbathing sessions of around 20 minutes at a time can do wonders for your mood, immunity, and vitamin D levels. If you live in a cloudy or winter-heavy region, consider supplementing with Vitamin D3/K2. If you're not already, everyone needs to be on Vitamin D3 according to the many doctors and experts I research. Modern lives call for more supplementation of certain things such as D3.
- Exercise will always be a foundational pillar of health, but if you're dealing with chronic illness or exercise intolerance, it's important not to overdo it. High cortisol from intense workouts can add more stress to your system. Instead, start with light activities like walking, yoga, qigong, and gentle mobility work.
- Even if you don't attend full classes for martial arts or exercise, make time to integrate some of the core techniques discussed earlier, such as squatting, hanging, pushups, or light calisthenics. Combine these with yoga stretches or Qigong meditation to create a daily practice that nourishes your body and mind.
- Above all, consistency is key. Lasting change comes not from intensity, but from showing up regularly. Try to find movement and activities that help you release stress while supporting your body and spirit in a healthy, sustainable way.

Chapter 11
The Story of Your Life

"Although the world is full of suffering, it is also full of the overcoming of it."
— *Helen Keller*

So, what makes the difference in people? What sets someone apart? What keeps a person moving forward while another remains stuck, or even spirals deeper into suffering? What allows some to overcome adversity while others struggle to find their way out? These are powerful questions worth taking time to reflect on for yourself. But as you consider them, allow me to offer a few prompts and pieces of wisdom to help guide your thinking.

To me what makes the difference is each person's Spirit. To me it's that fighting Spirit that keeps me going and kept me going when I was in those very dark places. Also, trust in that part of you, that spark. Like there's no other option, BUT to keep going, to keep searching, finding and questing. Trust that there's a deeper purpose guiding you, even if it's not yet clear. Let that belief propel you forward in your pursuit of happiness and inspire you every day.

There's nothing more important than living a healthy, fulfilling life. But I've been in a place where that felt nearly impossible, living with chronic illness and panic disorder. It can be deeply depressing, emotionally and physically exhausting, and even disabling at times. This is especially true when you have a full plate: single parenting, being overworked, raising children, or just trying to keep up with the demands of daily life.

I hope this book serves as a light, whether you're in a tunnel, in the dark season, or simply feeling lost. I remember feeling like I was deep in a cave, metaphorically speaking, looking up at a distant light. What struck me was that the light never disappeared. That's important. I came to understand that light as the strength of my Spirit. My soul never left me. And maybe there was even some kind of spiritual help there too. I don't know what that looks like for you, but for me, that light kept growing stronger and brighter. Some might call that *hope*.

There is always a way forward. There is always help. And there are always tools to add to your toolbox of life. I believe there's something greater than me that fuels that quiet, relentless drive to keep going. You can see it in certain people, the ones who radiate inner strength despite everything. When I see them, I think, "the Spirit is strong with that one."

Growing up without clear parental boundaries or consistent discipline can leave a child feeling emotionally unanchored, even if the intention was love, freedom, or gentleness. While nurturing and compassion are essential, structure and boundaries are just as vital for a child's healthy development, especially for the nervous system. Children need to know where the edges are, not just to feel safe, but to build an internal compass. Without those edges, the world can feel overwhelming, unpredictable, and emotionally unsafe. Too much gentle parenting, without firmness and guidance, can unintentionally create an inner world that lacks clarity, resilience, and self-regulation.

When a child isn't given consistent limits or consequences, the nervous system doesn't learn how to tolerate frustration, process discomfort, or navigate healthy authority. This can lead to emotional fragility, difficulty with self–discipline, and a body that's wired for anxiety or disassociation. Instead of growing up strong and centered, the individual may feel like life pushes them around mentally, emotionally, and even physically. They may lack the internal structure to face challenges, tolerate stress, or stand firm in relationships and decisions. Their fight–or–flight system may be triggered too easily, or they may default to freeze, collapse, or people–pleasing as a survival pattern.

But this is not a life sentence. With awareness and healing, you can begin to re-parent yourself. You can build the structure you didn't receive by creating your own healthy boundaries, developing routines, and gently training your nervous system to handle discomfort without breaking. Strength doesn't mean harshness; it means holding yourself with both compassion and clarity. Just like a tree needs both sunlight and strong roots, we need both softness and structure to grow. And even if you didn't get that balance as a child, you can give it to yourself now. That is the beauty of conscious healing: you get to become the steady, rooted presence your younger self never had.

A healthy sense of control is essential for emotional balance and healthy boundaries, especially when it comes to managing anxiety and maintaining a steady mind. While too much control can lead to rigidity and perfectionism, too little control often results in feeling overwhelmed, scattered, or emotionally unhinged. When the mind lacks structure or grounding, small stressors can feel enormous, and emotions can swing dramatically without a clear sense of direction. Just the word control can bring up uncomfortable thoughts.

This lack of internal control is often at the root of anxiety where the nervous system feels unsafe, and the mind is constantly scanning for danger or uncertainty. Developing healthy control isn't about suppressing emotions or micromanaging life, but rather about cultivating inner leadership, the ability to pause, regulate your breath, observe your thoughts, and choose a response rather than reacting impulsively. Simple daily routines, mindful movement, breathwork, and clear boundaries all help build this kind of control. Over time, they create a sense of inner containment, where the mind feels safe, the body feels steady, and emotions are allowed to flow without taking over. This kind of balanced control is what transforms reactivity into resilience.

> **IMPORTANT NOTE:**
> Someone who is or has been in anxiety and hypervigilance for a long time in their life might even feel a little anxious about *not* having anxiety anymore. That sounds counterintuitive at first but let me explain. For a long time, the brain and the body become addicted to this everyday stress, anxiety and hypervigilance. It becomes "normal." And in a way that becomes the "known," and ultimately this becomes a distorted level of safety. So, after years of this, going back to equilibrium of REAL safety and a peaceful existence, to your mind and body, this may seem like the "unknown." The unknown can sometimes feel scary and bring about anxiety. People can get addicted to everyday stress as well. It's one reason why we keep going back the same things that are causing the stress response in the first place. So, if you are a person that fits this scenario, then just be aware of this and don't let it discourage you. Keep going at a healthy pace that feels good to you.

Real Life Scenarios

Let's go over some practical things from this book and how it looks like in real life.

When experiencing a panic episode, the first and most important step is to calm the nervous system, to "put out the fire." Rather than immediately trying to analyze the situation or chase down the root cause, the body needs to be brought back to safety first. Think of panic as a fire alarm blaring throughout your system. This isn't the moment to fix the wiring; it's the time to quiet the alarm.

One powerful tool is Emotional Freedom Technique (EFT) or tapping. This involves gently tapping on specific points on the body, such as the forehead, face, chest, or the side of the hand, while acknowledging your emotions or saying simple affirmations. This technique can help discharge emotional energy, soothe the nervous system, and send a signal to the brain that you're safe. Similarly, deep diaphragmatic "balloon" breathing, where you inhale slowly into your belly and exhale even more slowly, stimulates the vagus nerve, which shifts the body out of fight–or–flight and into a parasympathetic, calm state. Long, steady exhales are particularly grounding.

Other vagus nerve techniques can be just as effective. These include splashing cold water on your face, humming, gargling, or slowly moving your eyes from side to side without turning your head. These simple practices calm the brain stem and help rewire the nervous system toward a sense of safety. Physical movement is also key, getting up and walking, stretching, or even shaking out your hands and arms can help burn off the excess adrenaline that often comes with anxiety.

Another underrated yet powerful method is self–soothing through gentle touch. Applying light pressure or massage to the belly, chest, forehead, jaw, or feet can bring immediate relief and connection back to the body. Try slowly rubbing your belly in circles or placing your hand over your heart and applying gentle pressure while breathing deeply.

Your internal dialogue also plays a big role. It helps to name what's happening: "my mind and body think I'm in danger right now, even though there may not actually be a threat." Unless you're genuinely in danger, this statement can help break the cycle of fear.

Some people even use humor or sarcasm to disarm the panic response, saying things like, "oh yes, clearly I'm in danger, while sipping tea in my kitchen." This can add just enough mental distance from the fear to help you regain clarity.

Another helpful example in this area is understanding the biological response your brain and body go through during an anxious moment. Whether it's triggered by a past trauma (like PTSD) or a real-time stressful event, the physiological response is often the same. One of the main systems involved is the HPA axis, (hypothalamic–pituitary–adrenal axis). When your brain perceives a threat, the hypothalamus signals the pituitary gland, which in turn sends a message to the adrenal glands to release stress hormones, primarily cortisol and adrenaline (epinephrine). These hormones prepare your body for survival, putting you into what's commonly known as the fight, flight, or freeze state. Your heart rate increases, your muscles tense, your digestion slows, and your mind becomes hyper focused on danger.

This response is a normal and healthy function of the body, it's designed to keep you alive. However, in cases of chronic anxiety or unresolved trauma, the system can become overactive or hypersensitive, reacting to perceived threats that may not be dangerous in the present moment. Here's a polished version of your text with smoother flow and clearer language:

A vital part of healing and self-awareness is learning to distinguish between a real-time stressful event and an old alarm system being reactivated by the nervous system. Once you can recognize the difference, you can begin using grounding tools to bring your body and mind back into balance. Over time, as this awareness deepens, you start to retrain how your system responds to stress. Some experts, including Michael from *PanicFree TV*, describe this process as a kind of rewiring, reclaiming balance in the nervous system. With consistent practice, when a real stressor does arise, the body still becomes alert, but the response is more calm, clear, and action-oriented, rather than being completely overtaken by a fight, flight, or freeze reaction. This is the shift from survival to resilience.

Tracking your symptoms with a 1–10 scale can also help ground you. Ask yourself, "what number am I right now?" This can reveal progress, even if small, such as going from a level 8 to a level 6, and gives your thinking mind a task that pulls it out of the emotional spiral.

Journaling, particularly using Socratic questioning (you read this in CBT Chapter 7), is another valuable practice. Write down your fearful thoughts, and then challenge them with questions like: is this thought actually true? What evidence supports or contradicts it? What would I say to a friend who was feeling this way? This builds emotional resilience over time and helps develop more balanced, grounded thinking.

Sometimes, nothing helps more than connection. Call or text someone you trust, not necessarily to fix the situation, but simply to be reminded that you're not alone. Even a short, caring interaction can signal safety to your nervous system. Lastly, close your eyes and think of something that brings you a sense of peace, whether it's a calming memory, a spiritual belief, a person you love, or a safe place. Visualizing safety can be a powerful anchor in the midst of panic situation.

Once the immediate panic has been calmed, the next step is addressing the root cause, the deeper patterns that keep the anxiety cycle going. This can be mentally difficult because you want to be able to work on this when you are calm and that can be tough since if you're anything like I was, I wasn't calm all that much. When I did find some peace, the last thing I wanted to do was bring up the very thing that "caused" the trigger and anxiety in the first place. It must be done, though, so you can finally heal and move through it so it doesn't affect you anymore, whatever it is.

This is where cognitive work becomes essential. Cognitive Behavioral Therapy (CBT) is a powerful tool for uncovering and challenging the limiting beliefs, cognitive biases, and distorted thought patterns that fuel anxiety. Many anxious thoughts are automatic and fear–based, often exaggerating danger or minimizing your ability to cope. Journaling with these patterns in mind, identifying them, questioning them, and rewriting them, can help retrain your mind to respond more rationally and compassionately over time.

Reaching out to a loved one can also help during this process, especially if they're someone who listens well and can help you reflect constructively. But for deeper healing, working with a qualified therapist can be incredibly valuable. I personally saw several therapists before I found one that truly fit. I had sessions with two different professionals, and while both offered something, neither felt quite right. I simply communicated that I wanted to try someone else, and the third therapist I saw was a much better match. That experience taught me something important: therapy is not one–size–fits–all and it's okay, even healthy, to advocate for what works best for you. This is part of building boundaries, honoring your needs, and taking ownership of your healing journey.

Let's walk through a real–life example of how to use these tools during a panic episode. Imagine you're at the grocery store. Everything seems fine, you're picking up produce or moving through the aisles, when suddenly, out of nowhere, a wave of panic hits. Your chest tightens, your heart races, and your thoughts start to spiral: *"I need to leave. Something's wrong."* Your body feels like it's in danger, even though nothing threatening is actually happening.

The first step is to put out the fire. You don't need to figure out why it's happening in the moment; you just need to calm your nervous system. So, you step aside to a quieter part of the store, find a place to pause, and begin using what you've practiced. You start with Emotional Freedom Technique (EFT). (Please find an EFT video for anxiety or panic and follow along anytime you start to feel this fight-flight-freeze response).

Next, you shift into deep diaphragmatic "balloon" breathing. You focus on slowly breathing into your belly, allowing it to expand like a balloon, and then exhaling even slower, aiming for a 4-second inhale and a 6-to-8-second exhale. This naturally stimulates your vagus nerve and begins to calm your entire system. You enhance this effect with a few vagus nerve techniques: a soft hum under your breath and slow, side–to–side eye movements to further settle your body. Your hands stop shaking, and your head feels clearer.

Still feeling that restlessness, you begin walking slowly through the aisle, using movement to help burn off the excess adrenaline. Even small steps help your body process the survival energy. At the same time, you place one hand gently on your chest and rub in slow, circular motions. Maybe you also massage your forehead or temples. These simple gestures are forms of self–soothing that bring comfort and remind your body that it's safe.

In the midst of it all, you start talking to yourself internally. You remind yourself, "my mind and body think I'm in danger right now, but I'm actually just here picking out vegetables." Maybe you even throw in a little humor or sarcasm, saying something like, "Oh no, the cabbage is going to attack me." Humor might seem silly in a moment like this, but it's a proven way to interrupt fear–based thinking and bring your brain back online.

You then do a quick check–in: "on a scale of 1 to 10, where am I?" You realize that when the panic first hit, it was a 9, but now it feels more like a 6. That small shift gives you a sense of progress and control. Later you can take a few minutes to journal. You ask yourself, "what was I afraid of? What triggered it? What thoughts did I have? What's the evidence that I was actually in danger?" This kind of Socratic questioning helps break the emotional hold of the panic and builds resilience over time.

Maybe after all that, you decide to call a friend, not necessarily to talk about the panic, but just to connect and hear a familiar, caring voice. That warmth and reassurance can be incredibly grounding. To close the loop, you take a quiet moment to visualize something that brings you comfort and safety, a memory, a person, a place. You let that image wash over you, settle into your body, and bring you back to center.

This is how these tools work, not in theory, but in real life. Not perfectly. Not instantly. But powerfully. With practice, you begin training your mind and body to respond differently. And soon, panic no longer runs the show, YOU do.

Panic often arises when the brain and body perceive a threat, whether that threat is real, imagined, or rooted in unhealed trauma from the past. For some, it begins with a sudden health sensation: a racing heart, dizziness, or shortness of breath. These bodily shifts, though often harmless, can trigger an overwhelming fear that something is seriously wrong, especially for those who have experienced medical scares or are highly attuned to their physical state. The body reacts as if in crisis, even when no danger is present.

Being in crowded or confined spaces, like packed buses, elevators, or concert halls, can also provoke panic. The mind may interpret these situations as inescapable, igniting a claustrophobic response and a need to flee. Similarly, the act of public speaking or being the center of attention can trigger a primal fear of judgment or rejection. For some, simply standing up in a meeting or introducing themselves can bring on symptoms of panic rooted in social anxiety.

Driving or riding in a car, particularly on highways or bridges, can be another major trigger. A past car accident, or simply the fear of losing control while moving at high speeds, can make what seems like a normal activity feel terrifying. Financial stress is also a common cause, unexpected bills, debt, or even just the thought of not having enough can flood the system with fear and overwhelm, especially if there's a history of scarcity or financial insecurity.

Relationship conflict or fear of abandonment can be another powerful source of panic. Whether it's an argument, a breakup, or the subtle fear that someone is pulling away emotionally, the nervous system may react as though the threat is life or death, especially for those with deep attachment wounds. Panic can also arise from substance-related causes, such as drinking too much caffeine, taking certain medications, experiencing alcohol withdrawal, or reacting to supplements that overstimulate the system. This is also part of nutrition and the body reacting or responding to nutritional deficiencies or toxins circulating in the body.

For those under intense work pressure, the constant push to meet deadlines, please others, or maintain a professional image can lead to perfectionism, imposter syndrome, and eventually panic. Even if the body is sitting still, the mind is racing to keep up with the fear of failure. Trauma triggers can also be subtle and unpredictable. A sound, smell, place, or even a word can unconsciously remind the body of a past traumatic event, causing a sudden flood of fear without a clear source.

Feeling trapped or powerless, such as being stuck in traffic, obligated to attend an event, or caught in a difficult life situation without clear solutions, can also lead to a panic response. The nervous system interprets this lack of control as dangerous. In other cases, long-term overstimulation, such as constant scrolling, noise, blue light exposure, and multi-tasking, can silently erode the brain's ability to regulate calm, eventually leading to emotional overwhelm.

Even something as simple as a lack of sleep or nutrient deficiency can weaken the body's resilience and lead to a heightened stress response. Over time, these small imbalances build up and lower the threshold for panic to set in. And for some, existential anxiety, such as fears about health, aging, death, or meaninglessness, can stir a deep and intense internal reaction, even if everything on the outside appears calm.

Each of these examples is rooted in the same pattern: the body is reacting to a perceived threat, trying to keep you safe. But when the system is overworked, inflamed, or carrying unresolved trauma, it often overreacts to situations that aren't truly dangerous. Understanding your own triggers and how your nervous system responds is the first step to healing. Panic is not weakness; it's a signal. With the right tools and self–awareness, you can learn how to listen, respond, and gradually regain your sense of calm and control.

Here are some examples of how to journal through a real–life situation, specifically when there is no immediate or obvious danger to your health or safety. Before you begin, always take a moment to pause and assess:

Is there a real threat right now? Am I in physical danger?

If there is a true emergency, seek help. But if you've already had appropriate medical testing or doctor visits and have ruled out serious health conditions, or have a clear understanding of them, then what you're likely experiencing is a panic situation, resistance emotionally to something, or your nervous system reacting to a perceived threat, not an actual one. This is where journaling, reflection, and grounding tools can help you regain a sense of calm and clarity. Just the simple act of writing or even typing in your phone can help to bring you out of the emotional part of the brain and into the logical side of the brain.

1. **Panic Trigger: Health Sensations (racing heart, shortness of breath, dizziness)**

   Scenario: I was sitting on the couch when I suddenly felt a flutter in my chest and a tightness in my breath. My heart started racing and my hands got cold.

   Put Out the Fire: I placed my hand over my chest, closed my eyes, and started balloon breathing, deep into the belly, slow on the exhale. I reminded myself, "This is just a body sensation. My body thinks I'm in danger, but I'm not." I started lightly tapping my collarbone (EFT), then stood up and walked slowly around the room, humming under my breath to calm my vagus nerve.

Journal Entry:
What am I feeling right now? Afraid. Like something's wrong with my heart.

Is this a real emergency? No. I've had this before. It always passes.

What's the evidence that I'm okay? I'm sitting at home, I'm not exerting myself, I've been checked out before, and this is a familiar pattern.

What would I say to a friend who feels this way? I'd say, "You're okay. Just breathe through it. Your body's on alert, but there's no fire. It will pass."

What number was it at its peak? 8 out of 10. Now? Maybe a 4. That's progress.

What do I need right now? To keep breathing, sip some water, and go outside for a few minutes.

2. **Panic Trigger: Crowded Space / Social Situation**

    Scenario: I was in a crowded grocery store, and suddenly I felt trapped, like I couldn't breathe. My vision narrowed, and I felt like I needed to escape.

    Put Out the Fire: I found a quiet corner by the carts and stood still. I began breathing deeply into my belly and slowly moved my eyes left and right. I lightly rubbed my sternum in circles and reminded myself, "This is just sensory overload. I've felt this before. It will pass." I even smiled softly to send a signal of safety to my brain.

Journal Entry:
What triggered me? Probably the noise, the lights, and the crowd, it felt like too much all at once.
Is the store dangerous? No. My brain just hit the overload button.
What thoughts came up? "I can't breathe." "I need to get out."

Are those thoughts true? No, I *am* breathing, and I stayed. I didn't run.

What would help next time? Go earlier in the morning. Listen to calming music while shopping. Take breaks if I need to.

How do I feel now? Lighter. Like I'm learning how to be with myself, even when it's hard.

3. **Panic Trigger: Conflict or Fear of Rejection (Relationship or Emotional Conflict)**

   Scenario: I had a tense conversation with someone I care about. After the call, my chest felt heavy, my stomach dropped, and I started spinning into panic, fearing they were pulling away or angry with me.

   Put Out the Fire: I sat with my feet on the floor, hand on my belly, and began deep breathing. I placed a hand over my heart and repeated slowly, "I am safe. I am okay. I can handle this." I stood up, shook out my arms, and did some light stretching while focusing on slow exhales.

Journal Entry:
What's the story in my head? "They're mad at me. I said the wrong thing. They're going to leave."

Is that true? No. They didn't say that. We had a disagreement, and that's normal.

What am I really afraid of? Being abandoned. Feeling unworthy.

What would I say to myself as a child? "You are loved even when things feel tense. Conflict doesn't mean rejection."

What's one kind thing I can do for myself now? Take a walk, make some tea, text a friend I trust.
How intense was the panic? It peaked at a 7. Now it's a 3. I rode the wave and it passed.

4. **Panic Trigger: Driving or Highway Anxiety**

   Scenario: I was merging onto the freeway when I suddenly felt overwhelmed. My palms got sweaty, my heart started pounding, and a wave of panic surged through me. I wanted to pull over immediately, but there was nowhere to stop.
   Put Out the Fire: I slowed down slightly and focused on deep belly breathing. I whispered to myself, "You're okay. You've driven this route before. This is just a wave." I kept my hands firmly on the wheel, turned down the radio, and focused on the car in front of me, staying present.

   Journal Entry:
   What was I afraid of? Losing control, crashing, or not being able to escape.

   Did that actually happen? No. I stayed on the road. I breathed through it and stayed present.

   What helped? Slowing down my breath, talking gently to myself, and staying focused on the road.

   What could I do next time? Remind myself before I drive that I have tools now. Maybe listen to calming music or a short grounding meditation beforehand.

   How do I feel now? Proud. A bit tired, but proud that I didn't let the fear take over.

5. **Panic Trigger: Work Deadline or Performance Pressure**

   Scenario: I opened my email and saw a last-minute project deadline. My chest tightened, my thoughts began racing, and I immediately felt like I wasn't going to be able to get it all done. I felt frozen and panicked, like I was failing before I even started.

Put Out the Fire: I stood up from my chair and walked to another room to break the loop. I started balloon breathing—inhale for 4, exhale for 8. I stretched my arms overhead and shook out the tension in my shoulders. I repeated, "It's just a deadline. I've handled harder things."

Journal Entry:
What story did my brain start telling me? "You're going to mess this up. You don't have enough time. You'll disappoint everyone."

Is that actually true? No. I've handled much more under pressure. I just need to take it one step at a time.

What am I really afraid of? Not being good enough. Being judged.

What helps? Breaking things into smaller tasks. Taking breaks to reset.

What will I do now? Write a short to–do list. Drink some water. Focus on just the first task.

6. Panic Trigger: Conflict at Home or Fear of Confrontation

Scenario: A small disagreement with a family member turned into a tense exchange. They raised their voice, and instantly I felt like I was shrinking inside—tight chest, flushed face, and the urge to run or shut down completely.

Put Out the Fire: I stepped outside, away from the energy of the moment. I placed one hand on my belly and one on my chest and focused on slow, rhythmic breathing. I reminded myself, "This is not the past. You are not trapped. You are safe now."

Journal Entry:
What was I reacting to? The tone of voice, the pressure, and my fear of confrontation.
What did my body feel? Like I was being attacked, even though it

was just a disagreement.

Is this the same as past experiences? It triggered old feelings, but this is a different situation, and I have tools now.

What would I tell my younger self in this moment? "You're allowed to pause. You're not in danger. You can respond when you're ready."

What helped me come down? Stepping outside, breathing, reminding myself that I'm allowed to take space.

7. Panic Trigger: War Veteran hears fireworks or similar sounds and has a PTSD Panic response.

Scenario: Walking the dog or outside somewhere and you hear a helicopter, or some kids let off fireworks, or a car starts to backfire.

Put Out the Fire: You bring up an EFT video on anxiety and panic and follow along with the video. This will help bring you into the logical side of your brain and out of the emotions. Try a few deep breathing exercises and some self-massage to activate the vagus nerve.

Journal Entry:
What was I reacting to? I realized it was just a couple of kids setting off the fireworks (or whatever it may be). My brain has a "stored file" of trauma that whenever there is a similar sound of fireworks, etc., my brain and body "think" there is a similar danger to when I was being shot at. I understand there is no danger now, and it's highly likely that I won't be shot at where I'm at in my life, so I want to start thinking about letting that fear go because it's a highly improbable event. (Unless this isn't true and you live in a war-torn area, etc.)

What did my body feel? My heart started to beat faster, and I started breathing faster. My mind started thinking of all the bad things that could happen and "what if's"? Sweating and clammy hands. 8/10

Is this the same as past experiences? This is NOT the same, the past was 180 degrees different. This was not a dangerous situation at all. *What would I tell my younger self in this moment?* Maybe I would say that having these responses isn't weakness, and that with hard work and fortitude I can overcome these events so they don't happen anymore. Doing alternative medicine and techniques is also very healthy and healing and I don't shy away from them. The toughest ex-special forces and CIA operatives can still come down with PTSD and anxiety.

What helped me come down? EFT helped me this time. Thinking and contemplating what was happening logically and reason helped understand and start to shift the triggered response. I'm going to keep doing this until the trigger response is fully discharged. I have the self-confidence to keep going.

Each of these journal entries highlights that while panic feels overwhelming in the moment, it can be navigated with the right tools and inner dialogue. The goal isn't perfection—it's progress. The more we learn to recognize, ground, and reflect, the more power we reclaim over how we respond to the world around us.

More Real-Life Examples:

I'd like to share a few more examples, in a more informal manner, of how I can help you navigate this process on a personal level.

Let's say a triggering event shows up. My first go-to action would be to have you splash cold water on your face. Stand up, move around a little—get some movement going. Let's say you're currently at an 8 out of 10 on the anxiety scale. If needed, grab a paper bag; that's perfectly fine. Your blood may need a little more CO_2 to balance out oxygen levels and help calm the body. Breathing into a paper bag helps with this.

Next, I'd have you use Emotional Freedom Technique (EFT), the same technique I shared earlier in the book. I highly recommend Brad Yates for this; he's one of the best, so there's no reason for me to reinvent the wheel. After about 10 minutes of EFT, the fire should start coming down. Let's say you go from an 8/10 to around a 4 or 5 out of 10—much more manageable.

Now, we check in with your breathing. Can you take a deep, full breath? Maybe not yet, because of the stress response. If needed, wait a little longer for things to come down further, perhaps to a 4 or 3 out of 10. Then try abdominal balloon breathing. Sit slightly leaning forward and work on expanding your belly as much as is comfortable. This stretches the diaphragm, pressing it downward and helping to stimulate the vagus nerve, which can activate the parasympathetic nervous system and bring more calm.

Let's backtrack: maybe you're at a 5 or 6 out of 10 and you're not ready for deep breathing yet. Instead, try more vagus nerve techniques. Splash cold water again on your face and neck. Grab an ice pack or cold compress and gently hold it to one side of your neck for about 20 seconds, then alternate. Do this for a couple of minutes while walking around the house. You might drop to 3 out of 10. From there, you could call a friend or loved one, someone who can help you feel connected. Maybe you're able to get a long, close hug and trigger a release of oxytocin. Now you're down to a 1 or 2 out of 10.

Here's another example: maybe you're at a 6 or 7 out of 10. You splash cold water, then go outside in the sunlight, get your bare feet on the ground (earthing), and maybe gargle some water or hum along to a song. The longer the exhale, the more this activates the vagus nerve and calms the heart. This alone might bring you down to a 3 or 4 out of 10, or maybe even a 0 or 1. You never know!

Or maybe you're in an anxious moment at a 6 out of 10, and all you do is have a calm internal dialogue. You pause and think, *"Hmm... I'm feeling anxiety right now. I wonder why? Oh—that's why."* Stay curious. Stay out of emotion as much as possible, and lean into the logical brain. *"Right now, my body thinks I'm in danger because my mind thinks there's danger. But is there real danger? No. I've already ruled that out. This is an irrational danger—just a panic false alarm."*

This type of self-talk helps signal your brain to stop triggering the adrenal glands to pump out more adrenaline. But the adrenaline that's already circulating needs to be burned off. That's when you go for a short walk, move up and down the stairs, or do some gentle exercise. This helps metabolize the catecholamines, the chemicals driving that fight–or–flight feeling. After moving, you might drop to a 2 out of 10, which is much easier to manage. An hour later, maybe you're back to 1 or even a 0.

Keep in mind that everyone is different. People have different constitutions, personalities, beliefs, and biases. No single tool works the same way for everyone. The key is to experiment, stay patient, and build your personal toolkit.

PanicFree TV

I took a course from Michael over at *PanicFree TV* years ago. Some of the techniques he teaches became powerful tools for me, which I still use. They've had a lasting impact, which is why I wanted to include them in this book. But I also chose to wait until the end, because in my opinion, they're more advanced. Now that you've worked through earlier chapters and hopefully built up a solid foundation of tools, habits, and awareness, I think you're ready to explore these deeper strategies. These aren't "quick fixes," but they're incredibly effective when applied consistently and with patience.

In his *PanicFree TV* course, Michael emphasizes a powerful advanced tool: identifying your panic triggers and proactively exposing yourself to them in a safe setting. You begin by carefully listing the thoughts, physical sensations, or situations that reliably evoke fear, rapid heartbeat, or unsettling "what–if" thoughts. Once you've made your list, choose one trigger to "activate" during a controlled, calm moment, such as at home, with supportive grounding tools by your side and without real danger present. This may feel uncomfortable at first, but the key is intentionally provoking a mild version of your trigger while remaining safe. By repeatedly doing this, the body and brain begin to learn that the trigger doesn't equal real danger, helping to "rewire" your nervous system and reduce the power these triggers hold over you.

Michael also highlights the importance of two counterintuitive strategies:
1. Reframe panic as a "false alarm." Your brain acting like an overly sensitive fire alarm, prioritizing safety by mistake, not attacking you. Recognizing panic this way reduces fear of panic itself.
2. Use paradoxical exposure, instead of fighting panic, deliberately invite it, like turning up the volume on the alarm. This unexpected confrontation often diffuses intensity, breaking the vicious cycle, whereas attempting to suppress panic, makes it worse. This is why I was writing earlier on about using sarcasm or cynicism. That might not be for everyone, but it's a great little trick that can help the brain switch from fight or flight or freeze, into a calmer state.

Trigger Awareness & Reflection Exercise:

Knowing and understanding your triggers is not about reliving your past. It's about reclaiming your power in the present. Take a few minutes in a calm space to gently reflect on things that tend to cause emotional distress, anxiety, or panic. These might be people, places, situations, or even certain memories, thoughts, or words. There is no right or wrong answer, just observe.

Common Trigger Examples:

Environmental or Situational Triggers:
- Loud, sudden noises (sirens, fireworks, yelling)
- Crowded spaces or traffic
- Medical settings or hospitals
- Being alone or confined
- Returning to a place where something painful happened

Emotional or Mental Triggers:
- Feeling out of control or trapped
- Intimacy or emotional closeness

- Being dismissed, ignored, or invalidated
- Unexpected change or pressure to make a quick decision
- Flashbacks of shame, fear, or guilt

Relational or Social Triggers:
- Arguments or raised voices
- Feeling judged or criticized
- Authority figures (bosses, police, etc.)
- Being gaslit or misunderstood
- Witnessing someone else in distress

Use the following worksheets to identify your personal triggers. I've included a few of them so you can see how your triggers change over time. You may also want to make notes about what has helped you work on your triggers so you can see how much progress you've made!

Your Personal Triggers

Take your time and fill these in at your own pace. You can always come back later and add more.

1. _____
2. _____
3. _____
4. _____
5. _____
6. _____
7. _____
8. _____
9. _____
10. _____

Remember: You are not defined by your triggers. Becoming aware of them is the first step in learning to manage and transform them.

Your Personal Triggers

Take your time and fill these in at your own pace. You can always come back later and add more.

1. _____
2. _____
3. _____
4. _____
5. _____
6. _____
7. _____
8. _____
9. _____
10. _____

Remember: You are not defined by your triggers. Becoming aware of them is the first step in learning to manage and transform them.

Your Personal Triggers

Take your time and fill these in at your own pace. You can always come back later and add more.

1. _____
2. _____
3. _____
4. _____
5. _____
6. _____
7. _____
8. _____
9. _____
10. _____

Remember: You are not defined by your triggers. Becoming aware of them is the first step in learning to manage and transform them.

Your Personal Triggers

Take your time and fill these in at your own pace. You can always come back later and add more.

1. _____
2. _____
3. _____
4. _____
5. _____
6. _____
7. _____
8. _____
9. _____
10. _____

Remember: You are not defined by your triggers. Becoming aware of them is the first step in learning to manage and transform them.

> **PANIC TO POTENTIAL TIP:**
> One surprisingly effective technique I've used and recommend, is using a bit of humor, sarcasm or light cynicism to talk back to anxiety when it shows up. It's like saying, "Oh, you again? Thought you'd show up eventually," or "Nice try, body. We've done this before. I'm not falling for it today." This approach helps reframe the moment. Rather than spiraling into fear, you're stepping into a place of calm confidence with a touch of humor. If you feel a wave of tension or unease, try saying, "Hmm, chest feels weird... must be Tuesday," or "Thanks for the awkward adrenaline boost. I didn't need coffee anyway." By treating the sensations or thoughts as a bit annoying rather than threatening, you take away their power. It signals to your brain that you're not in real danger, which can help settle the nervous system and prevent the spiral. It's a mindset shift, one that says: "I see you, I'm not impressed, and I'm moving on."

One of the last things I want to talk about is another list of foundational exercises for you. This way you have more and more examples to follow and support you. Let's go over these five here:

Grounding yourself in a safe place:

Find five things you can see. Look around and say them to yourself with some description. Find four things you can touch. Express what the item feels like by explaining them out loud. This feels smooth, flat, rough, cold, warm, sharp, squishy. Find three things you can hear. Listen to all the sounds going on, this might take a few moments, what's going on inside, outside, your breath, etc. Find two things you can smell. Your armpits and breath?! Find one thing you can taste. Go eat something and really pay attention to the tastes and smells.

> **PANIC TO POTENTIAL TIP:**
> Just as we went over in Chapter 7 on CBT, always remember to look at the **ABCDE of CBT.**

Controlled Exposure Therapy

These are all things you've read about already. Make sure you're in a safe place, and that you feel calm and relaxed in the body and mind. Think about one of your triggers and what would be the very first and easiest step to take towards overcoming that fear. For example, if you fear spiders, look at a photo of a spider, draw a picture of a spider, have someone hold a spider far away, watch a Spiderman movie, or have an expert hold a spider close to you. Over weeks of this, you may be able to get close to a spider without a triggering episode. Each time you engage with this exposure therapy, make sure you are ready to use the techniques we've talked about in this book for any incoming triggers.

Somatic Tracking

Find where the tension and pain are in your body. This is where yoga and other physical therapy and bodywork come into play. Do more work on those areas and try to release this tension. Breathe into the area. Focus on the area one at a time—where your attention goes, energy flows. Pain is usually some form of blockage, knotted up tissue and blood stagnation. Pain can be trauma, like a memory of that particular area. Self massage works great with Somatic work as well.

Narrative Reframing

Re-organize and contextualize the trauma. Change the story. Bring in understanding. This can be one of the most powerful root-cause healing techniques out there. Refer to Chapter 7 for more information.

1. **Identify the Current Narrative:** the first step is to recognize the existing story or perspective, including the emotions, beliefs, and interpretations associated with it.
7. **Challenge Assumptions:** question the assumptions and beliefs embedded in the current narrative. (Socratic thinking – ABCDE of CBT).
8. **Explore Alternative Perspectives:** consider different ways of understanding the situation, perhaps from the perspective of others or by focusing on different details or outcomes. (Talk Therapy with a professional, contemplative self-talk and journaling).
9. **Reconstruct the Narrative:** re-author the story by incorporating new perspectives, reframing negative aspects into positive ones, and finding meaning and purpose in the experience.

IMPORTANT NOTE:
Here are a few things that I want to mention that I won't be going into or going over in this book, but I think are important to mention. These are intended for you to research on your own, but I wanted to make sure and talk about them because they are things I've read about that have helped people with PTSD, chronic anxiety and burnout.

Neurofeedback

Neurofeedback is a form of biofeedback (also called EEG biofeedback). This is a non-invasive technique that trains your brain to regulate itself more effectively by giving you real-time feedback on your brainwave patterns. During a session, sensors placed on your scalp measure electrical activity in targeted brain regions. That activity is then translated into simple visual or auditory cues, like a soundtrack that becomes clearer when your brain calms or a game that progresses when your focus steadies.

Over repeated sessions, your nervous system "learns" healthier patterns of arousal and self-regulation. For people with PTSD, anxiety, depression or attention-related challenges, neurofeedback can help reduce PTSD, hypervigilance, improve sleep, and enhance emotional resilience by directly strengthening the brain's ability to shift out of fight-flight-freeze modes and into more balanced states. I was talking with a friend who's been diagnosed with C-PTSD, and she's adopted this method wholeheartedly. She swears it's made a world of difference and has profoundly improved her life.

CGM – Constant Glucose Monitor

This device involves wearing a small patch on your arm that tracks your glucose levels in real time throughout the day, sending data directly to an app. While it can be a bit pricey, many people have found it incredibly helpful for understanding how blood sugar fluctuations affect mood, anxiety, and overall stress response. Personally, I haven't used one yet, mostly because I'm currently following the GAPS diet and a zero–sugar, zero–carb lifestyle, but I do plan to try it in the future.

Hyperbaric Chamber

This involves sitting in a pressurized chamber while breathing pure oxygen. It's been shown to increase oxygen flow to the brain and body, support neurological repair, and reduce inflammation. Some studies suggest 'HBOT' may help ease symptoms of PTSD, anxiety, and even brain fog by calming the nervous system and promoting healing at the cellular level.

Applied Kinesiology

Also known as muscle testing, this technique involves assessing the body's response to various stimuli or questions through subtle changes in muscle strength. There are many variations of this method, and while it may seem unconventional to some, I've personally used self–testing for over a decade and found it to be an insightful tool when done properly. I highly recommend learning it under the guidance of someone who is truly experienced, ideally a practitioner who uses it professionally and with integrity.

Lymphatic Drainage

I've done some lymph drainage, and it definitely helps detoxification, which is much needed in this modern world where we are bombarded with toxins daily.

Lymphatic drainage is a vital yet often overlooked aspect of our body's natural detoxification system. Unlike blood, which is pumped by the heart, lymph must be moved through the vessels by the gentle contraction and relaxation of surrounding muscles and tissues. That means regular movement, whether through walking, yoga, light calisthenics, or even dedicated lymphatic exercises. This helps keep the lymph flowing freely, preventing stagnation and supporting immune health.

For those living with chronic illness, reducing lymph congestion can ease inflammation and discomfort, and may even have a calming effect on the nervous system, alleviating anxiety. I've used regular movement and simple self–massage techniques, such as gentle strokes toward the heart and dry brushing, which can further stimulate lymphatic flow. By integrating these practices into your daily routine, you'll be giving your body's built–in cleansing pathways the support it needs to function at its best.

MDMA - Psilocybin - Ketamine - Ibogaine

IMPORTANT NOTE:
Never engage in the use of psychedelic or psychoactive substances without proper medical supervision or guidance from a trained professional in a legal and safe setting. These substances can have powerful psychological effects and are not to be taken lightly. If explored, they should be done under the care of a qualified practitioner or licensed facility to ensure safety, integration, and support throughout the process.

There is a growing body of legitimate research in science, psychiatry, and trauma therapy exploring the use of psychedelic compounds—such as MDMA, ketamine, Ibogaine and psilocybin—for the treatment of PTSD and complex trauma. While I won't be covering these therapies here, I encourage you to follow developments in this field if it resonates with you. Under proper clinical supervision, many people have reported profound healing through these approaches.

Emotion Code

This is a fascinating healing modality that blends elements of Chinese medicine, psychology, and kinesiology. I personally enjoy working with it and use it often in my practice. While I won't be diving into the specifics of Emotion Code in this book, I felt it was important to mention because it has played a valuable role in my own healing journey. I continue to use it with clients, loved ones, and occasionally for myself when needed.

Theta Healing – "Woo–Woo Alert"

This is another powerful method I've found meaningful. Like Emotion Code, I won't be covering it in detail here, but it remains a regular part of my personal and professional toolkit. Theta healing works at a deep subconscious and energetic level and often requires one–on–one instruction and plenty of practice to fully grasp and apply.

In my experience, finding a skilled and grounded practitioner can make all the difference, as the quality of guidance is essential when working with such subtle and profound techniques.

Again, the above are simply tools I've come across or used in my own path. They are not one–size–fits–all solutions, but they may open a door to deeper healing when explored safely and intentionally.

In line with Theta Healing, I want to share some last thoughts on a very "woo–woo up in the clouds" knowledge and wisdom. If this is too far for you, please just skip ahead or skim through it. This was very meaningful to me in my life, which is why I'm sharing it, but it might not resonate with you.

Some of these so–called "masters" I encountered likely claimed to be something they weren't, but I took the knowledge and wisdom they shared and ran with it, so to speak.

Throughout my journey, I've studied with and spoken to Grandmasters, Shamans, Master Healers, and many types of spiritual practitioners. And yes, there is *very real substance* to these people, their roles, and the wisdom they carry.

Some of the people I've learned from devoted their entire lives to monkhood or the path of self–mastery, true practitioners of the craft. I've had the honor of studying with monks from the Shaolin Temple in China, a QiGong Kung Fu Grandmaster, and a Hawaiian Shaman who genuinely lived and breathed the tradition for most of his life. I also spent time with a Shaman in Mt. Shasta, yes, he was a little crazy and eccentric, but I wasn't there to judge, I was there to learn. There was more I won't go into, but these are just a few of the unique individuals who crossed my path, each with their own flavor of wisdom and experience.

These are spiritual and energetic healing tools, and if you feel called to go deeper into this realm, I highly recommend working with a skilled spiritual healer. That said, not everyone is wired for this kind of work, and that's perfectly okay. If you're sensitive to energy, it doesn't make you more or less special, or more or less "weird." Just like some people can handle more alcohol than others, it's not better or worse, just different.

Even the average person can develop the ability to sense energy and become more intuitive with time and practice. But here's my honest take, if you live a typical Western lifestyle with modern responsibilities, diving deeply into energetic healing, lightwork, or shamanism can sometimes be destabilizing. It's not something to casually mix with a 9–5 life, parenting, or the constant buzz of modern living. Shamans, monks, and master healers usually live temple or retreat–style lives for a reason—this path asks a lot of you.

The beliefs listed below can also simply reflect mental and emotional limitations, not just spiritual ones. Often, they can be explored and worked through using Cognitive Behavioral Therapy (CBT) or other therapeutic tools—just some food for thought as you reflect on your healing journey.

Common Healer '*Oaths & Vows*' That May Be Limiting You:

Vow of Poverty
- "I must not charge for healing work."
- "True healing should always be free."

These beliefs can block financial flow and create guilt around abundance.

Vow of Self–Sacrifice
- "Others come first, always."
- "My needs don't matter if others are suffering."

These beliefs can lead to burnout, neglect of self–care, and codependency.

Vow of Silence
- "It's not safe to speak my truth."
- "I will be persecuted if I share my healing gifts."

These beliefs often stem from trauma (sometimes ancestral or past life), and can suppress expression, voice, and spiritual teaching.

Oath to Take on the Pain of Others
- "Let me absorb their pain so they don't have to suffer."
- "I'll carry their burden for them."

These beliefs can create energetic overwhelm, chronic fatigue, and emotional entanglement.

Vow of Humility or Invisibility
- "I must stay hidden or small to remain spiritually pure."
- "If I become successful or visible, I'll lose my power."

These beliefs can block personal growth, visibility, and leadership.

Oath of Celibacy or Emotional Detachment
- "I can't have romantic relationships and be a healer."
- "Emotions cloud spiritual wisdom."

These beliefs can prevent intimacy, joy, and full embodiment.

Vow to Heal Everyone, No Matter the Cost
- "It's my duty to help everyone who asks, even if it hurts me."

These beliefs can lead to exhaustion, resentment, and healer martyrdom.

Oath of Obedience to a Tradition or Lineage
- "I must only do things the way my teacher or lineage taught."
- "It's wrong to innovate or adapt spiritual practices."

These beliefs can lock intuition, evolution, and personal spiritual authority.

Vow of Perfection
- "I must be completely healed before I help others."
- "If I make a mistake, I'm not worthy of being a guide."

These beliefs can fuel imposter syndrome and delay sharing your gifts.

Oath of Isolation
- "I must walk this path alone."
- "No one will understand me."
-

These beliefs can prevent building community, support systems, and collaboration.

These vows can often be cleared through:
- Energy healing sessions (Emotion Code, Theta Healing, Reiki, etc.)
- Journaling and intention setting
- Exploring past life or inner child work
- Speaking new affirmations aloud:
    - "I release any vow, oath, or agreement that no longer serves me."
    - "I allow abundance, connection, and joy as a healer in this lifetime."

Angelic and Spiritual Healing

> **IMPORTANT NOTE:**
> Many Spiritual traditions, and something I've been told personally through my studies and experiences, teach that every human being has at least one guardian angel assigned to them for the entire duration of their physical life. This guardian angel watches over, protects, and gently guides us, often in subtle ways. Whether or not you've ever felt this presence consciously, the support is

always there, offering assistance, encouragement, and protection throughout your journey.

This concept isn't tied to any one religion, it's a universal idea that transcends belief systems. You don't need special training to connect with your guardian angel; just speaking from the heart, setting the intention, or even silently asking for guidance is enough to open the door to that support. Sometimes it's the whisper of intuition or the unseen hand that nudges you in the right direction when you need it most.

Working with angels, especially archangels, can bring a powerful sense of comfort, protection, and divine guidance. Many people experience deep emotional and energetic healing when calling upon specific archangels:

- **Archangel Michael** – For protection, strength, and cutting energetic cords.
- **Archangel Raphael** – For physical healing, emotional support, and restoring balance.
- **Archangel Gabriel** – For communication, clarity, and expression of truth.
- **Archangel Uriel** – For wisdom, insight, and illumination in times of confusion.

These energies are accessible to all who sincerely ask for help. Healing with angels often comes through visualization, prayer, intuitive impressions, or simply sensing their presence during meditation or difficult moments.

Ascended Master Connection

Ascended Masters are enlightened beings who once walked the earth in physical form and have since transcended, becoming spiritual guides and teachers from higher planes. This includes figures like:

- **Jesus (Yeshua/Christ Consciousness)** – Offering unconditional love, forgiveness, healing, and spiritual awakening.
- **Buddha** – Supporting mindfulness, inner peace, and the release

of suffering.
- **Quan Yin** – Representing compassion, grace, and gentle strength.
- **Saint Germain** – Known for transmutation and spiritual alchemy.
- **And others, whoever you feel best connecting to**

Many people feel drawn to one or more of these figures (including others not listed above) during their healing journey. You don't need to "worship" or even fully understand them to receive their support. Simply being open-hearted and respectful allows you to connect.

These spiritual beings can assist in lifting heavy emotional energy, deepening your intuition, and reconnecting you with your soul's path. Whether through meditation, prayer, journaling, or visualization, connecting to these higher frequencies can bring profound shifts in healing, insight, and spiritual growth.

The Story of Your Life

So, what comes next? That's up to you... I can lead you to water, but I can't make you drink. This is your life. Let the practices you've learned meet you where you are. Take what resonates, leave what doesn't, and keep going. You are not behind. You are not broken. You are in process.

At the end of the day, don't get stuck in the weeds. Try not to obsess over every little symptom or theory. Keep moving forward with your life while you work on the problems. Put out the immediate fires, chip away at the root causes, and keep taking sensible steps. If you get lost in endless processing or become fanatical about every tiny detail, it can actually spiral you backward. Progress is made by steady, practical action, not perfectionism.

You need a healthy dose of control, not rigid control that closes you down, but logical, rational, action-oriented control that helps your mind and body stabilize. After long periods of dysregulation, your nervous system has often been running wild. Bringing structure, routine, and small measurable habits back into your life gives your system a chance to reset. Move from reactive chaos into calm, deliberate choices.

There's room to let go and allow things to unfold, but trauma and PTSD often create too much "Yin," too much passivity, withdrawal, and avoidance. Balance requires a bit of "Yang," clear, consistent effort to manage your emotions and rebuild capacity. Take action, but don't rage against yourself for not being "fixed" overnight. Grounded, steady work wins the race. Keep it practical. Breathe. Prioritize. Do one useful thing each day. Over time, those small wins become the life you actually want to live.

IMPORTANT NOTE:
There's a fine line between pushing through fear and being brave. Just taking a step back to think things through first is a good strategy. Sometimes it's not about forcing yourself forward. It's about knowing what feels right for you, your constitution, your energy, and your personality.

Real courage can be either moving ahead or it can just be hitting pause to figure out the smartest move for where you're at. It's about finding that balance. For me, I felt that fear and anxiety when confronted with making decisions, whether to go left or right at the fork in the road. Even though I felt a lot of fear towards a certain decision, I did it anyway. Was it the right one? Looking back, without going into specific details, I can tell you that certain decisions, even though there was fear, were good decisions.

Others, when confronted with fears, may have found it best to get another opinion, ask for support, sleep on it and/or ask more questions. But, with me being in a state of hypervigilance, I couldn't wait. I couldn't sit still. I couldn't think very well. So, ask loved ones for their wisdom, write a pros and cons list, ask questions, get clarity and gather as much info or data on the situation. Most importantly, give yourself a backup, whatever that means for you. There was a time that I wanted to burn all my bridges, but needless to say, I won't be here to tell you to do that because after doing the work, I didn't need to.

If you've made it this far, I want to honor and congratulate you. Whether you read every chapter or simply followed your curiosity through certain parts, you've shown up for yourself, and that's no small thing. Healing from PTSD, chronic illness, anxiety, or burnout is achievable and usually isn't a straight path. It's a layered, often messy, deeply personal journey. But, one thing is certain: by becoming more aware of your body, thoughts, and energy, you're already on the path to change.

Healing isn't about fixing what's broken. It's about learning to listen to the signals your body and mind are sending you, sometimes softly, sometimes loudly, and responding with care. It's about building a new relationship with yourself based on trust, gentleness, and truth. There is no magic bullet or quick fix, but there is a way forward, and it's made up of small, consistent choices that begin to restore safety, balance, and vitality. I personally think the information in this book IS the shortcut and the "cheat codes" that people are looking for. There's more out there, some that none of us can imagine right now. So, stay open and free in your mind for things to unfold in the way that is best for you.

You now have tools. Whether it's breathwork, grounding exercises, self-massage, journaling, nervous system techniques, nutritional strategies, knowledge and information, psychology, and more, you've started to build a toolbox that can support you in real time. These aren't one-time fixes, they're living practices. Over time, they become like roots that keep you steady even when life brings stress or uncertainty.

You may still have days when the old patterns return. That's okay. That's human. You may even have some anxiety about not having anxiety anymore. I did…This process isn't about perfection; it's about cultivating a new baseline where your system can return to calm more easily, where you feel less hijacked by fear, and more in touch with your own power. There will be setbacks. But, there will also be breakthroughs, moments of clarity, new trust in your mind and body, and growing evidence that you are coming back to balance and homeostasis.

If there's one thing I hope you carry with you from this book, it's this: you are not alone, and there is a way through. The spark within you, the part of you that reached for this book in the first place is real, strong, and still here. And with every breath, every step, and every act of self–care, you are moving closer to the life you were always meant to live.

Because I am…

Takeaways from Chapter 11:

- It's time to truly start living your life, not trapped in an anxious bubble. No one is meant to exist in a constant state of fear or survival.
- Continue strengthening your healthy boundaries but be mindful of going to extremes that might isolate you from your social world. Balance is key.
- Control isn't the enemy. When used wisely and with self-awareness, it can be a powerful tool for creating stability and safety.
- Pay attention to the steps you can take immediately after a triggering or activating event. These are the moments where calming the "fire" is most effective.
- Learn to view the biological cascade of fight, flight, or freeze as information. It can serve as a tool to ground you and bring your mind back to the present.
- Acknowledge the process of healing the deeper roots of PTSD and the stress response. This work takes time, but awareness of the pattern is a powerful start.
- Remember, there are many other techniques available, as mentioned in this chapter, so if one speaks to you or feels aligned, don't hesitate to explore it further.
- Some people carry unconscious oaths or vows, like beliefs around self-sacrifice, staying small, or always putting others first. These can simply be **mental or emotional limitations**, not just spiritual. Reflecting on and releasing them can be a powerful step toward healing.
- We also explored the idea of connecting with **spiritual support**, such as angels or ascended masters as a source of comfort, strength, and higher guidance, if it resonates with you.

Author's Information:

Website: All go to the same site -- www.FromPanicToPotential.com -- www.Wasenshido.Org -- www.YogiWarriors.org

YouTube: @Wasenshido
Facebook: FarrenTayler
Instagram: @Wasenshido – Farren Tayler
Email: FarrenTayler@Gmail.com

Suggested Experts & Resources

Below is a curated list of experts, practitioners, and thought leaders whose work has informed and inspired much of the content in this book. I encourage readers to explore these resources independently to deepen their understanding of healing, wellness, and personal growth.

Medical Doctors & Functional Medicine Experts:

Dr. Michael Ruscio – Functional Medicine, Gut Health
Dr. Pradip Jamnadas – Cardiologist, Internal Medicine
Dr. Suneel Dhand – Internal Medicine Physician
Dr. Natasha Campbell–McBride – Neurosurgeon, Nutritionist, GAPS Diet
Dr. Stephen Hussey – Cardiovascular Health, Functional Medicine
Dr. William Davis – Cardiologist, Wheat Belly Author
Dr. Peter Osborne – Autoimmunity and Nutrition
Dr. Aseem Malhotra – Cardiologist, Public Health Advocate
Dr. Tony Hampton – Family Physician, Carnivore and Metabolic Health
Dr. Eric Berg – Health Educator, Nutrition and Keto
Dr. Ken Berry – MD, Low–Carb Advocate

Dr. Steven Gundry – Cardiologist, Heart Surgeon, Author
Dr. Sten Ekberg – Holistic Health and Metabolism
Dr. Darren Schmidt – Functional Medicine
Dr. Malcolm Kendrick – Heart Disease Research and Public Health
Dr. Paul Mason – Cholesterol and Low–Carb Expert
Dr. Nathan Bryan – Nitric Oxide Researcher
Dr. Eric Westman – Obesity, Metabolic Health
Dr. Marianne Teitelbaum – Ayurvedic and Chiropractic Practitioner
Dr. David Perlmutter – Neurologist, Brain Health, Uric Acid
Dr William Li – World-renowned Medical Physician, Scientist, Author
Dr Andrew Kutnik – PHD
Dr. David Rabin – Neuroscience and Wearable Technology
Dr. Thomas Seyfried – Cancer Research and Metabolism
Dr. Ford Brewer – Preventive Medicine, Lipidology
Dr. Ross Hauser – Regenerative Medicine
Dr. Shawn Baker – MD, Carnivore Diet Advocate
Dr. Mark Hyman – Functional Medicine, Public Health
Dr. Annette Bosworth (Dr. Boz) – Internal Medicine, Metabolic Health
Dr. Jeremy London – Heart Surgeon

Nutrition Scientists & Wellness Researchers:

Dr. Rhonda Patrick – Micronutrients, Longevity
Dr. Anthony Jay – Genetics, Hormones, Estrogenics
Dr. Robert Lustig – Sugar and Public Health
Dr. Paul Saladino – Carnivore Diet and Functional Medicine
Dr. Anthony Chaffee – Neurosurgery and Carnivore Advocacy
Dr. Ben Bikman – Insulin Resistance and Mitochondrial Function
Dr. Derrick Lonsdale – Thiamine (Vitamin B1) Research
Dr. Chris Masterjohn – Nutritional Biochemistry, Vitamin Research
Elliot Overton – Functional Nutritionist, Vitamin B1 Focus
Gary Brecka – Longevity, Biometrics, and Biohacking
Mike Mutzel – Functional Medicine, Gut–Brain Axis
Mary Ruddick – Nutritional Therapist, Gut Health
Barbara O'Neill – Natural Health and Detoxification

Mental Health, Psychology & Trauma Experts:

Dr. Bessel van der Kolk – Trauma Research, author of *The Body Keeps the Score*
Dr. Andrew Huberman – Neuroscience, Psychology, Lifestyle Habits
Dr. Jordan Peterson – Psychology, Behavior, Cultural Insight
Dr. Dawn Elise Snipes – Mental Health and CBT Educator
Patrick Teahan – Family Systems and Trauma Therapist
Kain Ramsay – Udemy Courses – Psychology and Personal Development

---

Public Educators, Creators & YouTube Channels:

Michael – *PanicFree TV*
Brad Yates – EFT Specialist (YouTube)
YOGABODY – Yoga, Mobility, Breathwork (YouTube)
Jesse Taylor – Martial Arts, Movement, and Mindfulness (YouTube)
Steak and Butter Gal – Carnivore Diet and Support (YouTube)

Psychology & Emotional Healing Experts:

Bessel Van Der Kolk, M.D. - Bessel van der Kolk is a Boston-based Dutch-American psychiatrist, author, researcher and educator. Since the 1970s his research has been in the area of post-traumatic stress. He is the author of four books, including The New York Times best seller, The Body Keeps the Score.

Milton Hyland Erickson -
American psychiatrist and psychologist specializing in medical hypnosis and family therapy. He was the founding president of the American Society for Clinical Hypnosis.

Antonio Damasio - A neuroscientist known for his groundbreaking work on the connection between emotion, reason, and the body. Author of *Descartes' Error: Emotion, Reason, and the Human Brain*,

The Feeling of What Happens, and *Self Comes to Mind.*

Paul Ekman - A pioneer in the study of facial expressions and emotions, especially how emotions are communicated nonverbally across cultures. Author of *Emotions Revealed, Telling Lies,* and *Unmasking the Face* (co-authored with Wallace V. Friesen).

Robert Plutchik - Best known for developing the Wheel of Emotions and his psychoevolutionary theory of emotion. Author of *Emotion: A Psychoevolutionary Synthesis* and *The Emotions: Facts, Theories, and a New Model*

Joseph LeDoux - A neuroscientist specializing in survival circuits in the brain, particularly those related to fear and anxiety. Author of *The Emotional Brain, Anxious: Using the Brain to Understand and Treat Fear and Anxiety* and *Synaptic Self.*

Lisa Feldman Barrett - A psychologist and neuroscientist who challenges traditional theories of emotion with a modern, brain-based perspective. Author of *How Emotions Are Made* and *Seven and a Half Lessons About the Brain.*

www.ingramcontent.com/pod-product-compliance
Lightning Source LLC
Chambersburg PA
CBHW020531030426
42337CB00013B/809